THE BOOK OF MEMORY

Also by Mark Rowlands

The Happiness of Dogs: Why the Unexamined Life is Most Worth Living

A Good Life: Philosophy from Cradle to Grave

Running with the Pack: Thoughts from the Road on Meaning and Mortality

The Philosopher and the Wolf: Lessons from the Wild on Love, Death and Happiness

THE BOOK OF MEMORY

How We Become Who We Are

MARK ROWLANDS

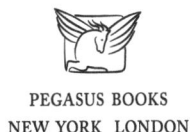

PEGASUS BOOKS
NEW YORK LONDON

THE BOOK OF MEMORY

Pegasus Books, Ltd.
148 West 37th Street, 13th Floor
New York, NY 10018

Copyright © 2025 by Mark Rowlands

First Pegasus Books cloth edition October 2025

All rights reserved. No part of this book may be reproduced in whole or in part without written permission from the publisher, except by reviewers who may quote brief excerpts in connection with a review in a newspaper, magazine, or electronic publication; nor may any part of this book be reproduced, stored in a retrieval system, or transmitted in any form or by any means electronic, mechanical, photocopying, recording, or other, or used to train generative artificial intelligence (AI) technologies, without written permission from the publisher.

ISBN: 978-1-63936-975-1

10 9 8 7 6 5 4 3 2 1

Printed in the United States of America
Distributed by Simon & Schuster
www.pegasusbooks.com

For Emma

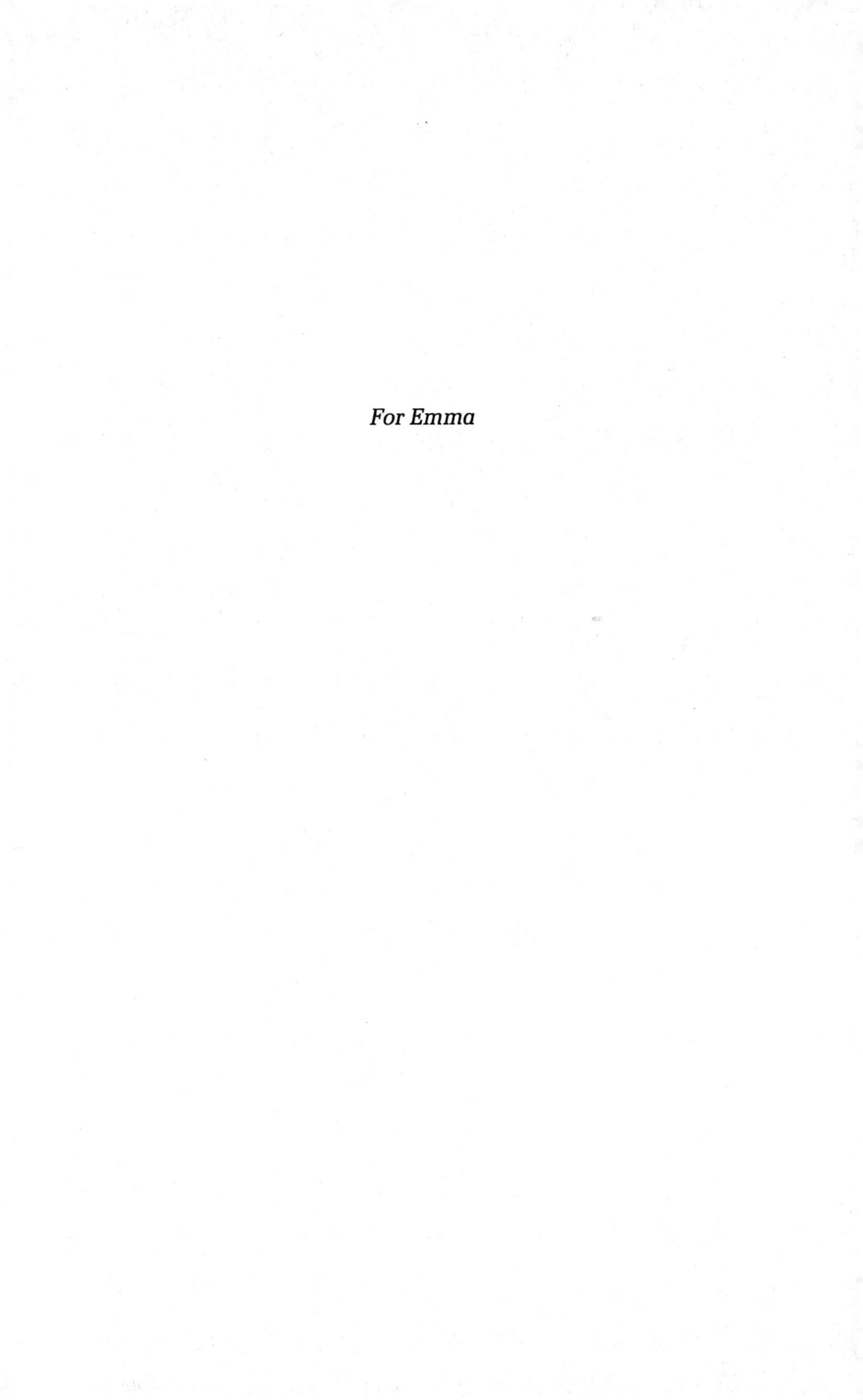

CONTENTS

Preface: My Life as a Fictional Character   1

PART ONE: THE BOOK OF MEMORY

1. The Path Out of the Woods   15
2. Second Chances   18
3. Metaphors   21
4. Kinds of Remembering   25
5. Highly Superior and Severely Deficient   30
6. The Book of You   35

PART TWO: THE WATERS OF LETHE

7. Patrick   43
8. Rilkean Memories   46
9. A Wake-up Call on Wimbledon Common   51
10. Home, Again   56
11. The Riverbank   60
12. Rilkean Style   65

PART THREE: BRIGHT ISLANDS IN THE NIGHT

13. Stendhal's Syndrome   73
14. *Challenger*   76
15. Making and Remaking Memories   80
16. The Beaches of Memory   85
17. Invitations   89
18. The Face of My Father   95

PART FOUR: NEGOTIATING WITH THE PAST

19. Earthquake   107
20. Super Piece of Cricket, That!   114
21. The Face of My Father, Redux   118
22. Ownership and Authorship in Memory   122
23. Miracles   127
24. So Long, Suckers!   131

Postface: My Afterlife as a Fictional Character   135

Further Reading   141
Acknowledgements   147

Preface

MY LIFE AS A FICTIONAL CHARACTER

'Life,' the playwright Tennessee Williams once claimed, 'is all memory, except for the one present moment that goes by so quick you can hardly catch it going.' Mrs Goforth, in whose mouth Williams put these words, may be right. Some people advocate living in the 'now', in this one present moment that is so hard to catch. But what is the 'now' other than an imaginary point built from recollections of the past and anticipations of the future – merely a shifting, notional line between what has been and what will be? The future, however, does not yet exist. It is merely a promise, diaphanous, insubstantial and unreliable, as many promises tend to be. But, we might think, the past has the solidity and substantiality of what has been written. All your piety and wit cannot call it back to cancel half a line. Fate can take away your future. But no matter what it does to you, it can never take away your past: the things you have done and the choices you have made. These acts and choices are written and can never be erased. When the universe eventually becomes a void – cold, dark and unbroken – it will still be true that once upon a time there was a person who made these choices and did these things, and that person was you.

The past, then: is that where you are to be found? If the past is more substantial than the light-as-a-feather future, then perhaps it would also be more real, as a flesh, blood and bone human being is more real than their ghost? After all, what could make you the person you are, on this pathway through space and time that is your life, other than the things you have witnessed, the things you have done, and the things that have happened to you? But these things are all creatures of the past. They no longer exist and are retained through memory. It is memory, therefore, that makes you who you are. Perhaps life is indeed all memory? And so too are you? Perhaps. I don't think any of these foregoing claims are untrue per se. But they are helpful only if we understand what memory is.

What if everything we thought we knew about memory is wrong? What if memory does not capture the past? What if the moving hand of the now can indeed be enticed backwards in time, to not only cancel lines but rewrite them at will? What if memory need not bind us to our past but can just as easily take us further away from it? What if a person's memory can live on in the mind of someone else? These are not idle 'what ifs'. As we shall see in the pages to follow, I

MY LIFE AS A FICTIONAL CHARACTER

think the safest general characterization of the tenor and direction of research in the science of memory over the preceding decades is that almost everything we thought we knew about memory is wrong. These 'what ifs' serve to highlight some of the dimensions of our error, and they are deeply intertwined. Collectively these errors herald new possibilities, glittering and hitherto undreamed of. At the core of these possibilities lies a truth: we are not what we thought we are. Our existential solidity is more imagined than real. We are, perhaps above all, and in a sense that this book will try to make clear, *genre confused*. The gap between us and fictional characters is not the vast chasm we have thought. There is a touch of the fictional about each one of us. In this truth, if one knows how to look, one can find salvation. Not, sadly, the possibility of life everlasting, but, nonetheless, a certain, more modest, way of escaping the prison walls of our births and deaths. If you want to know how I managed to cheat death – long before he made his grim appointment with me – please read on.

When we think about the difference between fiction and reality, the notion of truth is likely to make an early appearance in our thoughts. Works of fiction, we assume, share a common trait: they are not true. There never really was a Sherlock Holmes who lived on Baker Street and solved crimes. The claim that there was would be untrue. This absence of truth, many think, decisively distinguishes the fictional from 'the real'. That works of fiction are not true is, of course, definitional – it is what makes them fiction – but, nevertheless, it is not as straightforward as it may appear. After all, within fiction itself are both truths and falsehoods. Sherlock Holmes lived at 221B Baker Street. Within the collection of stories that make up the Sherlock Holmes corpus, this claim is true and the claim that he lived at 222 Baker Street is, accordingly, false. This sense of truth is internal to the stories. It is the failure of fiction to correspond to what we call the 'real' world – an external comparison of fiction with something that lies outside it – that underlies the idea that fiction is untrue. This sense of untruth, however, derives from another, deeper, feature of fiction: what is true – in the internal sense – of any fictional character depends entirely on what someone or other has written about them. Their existence is, in this sense, a *dependent* one – hinging entirely on the creative efforts of a writer.

If Conan Doyle wrote that Sherlock Holmes lived at 221B Baker Street, then that is enough to make it so, internally. Conan Doyle could have had Holmes live somewhere else, but he didn't. If I am an author writing about a fictional character that I have created, then I can, in essence, write whatever I like. There might be some constraints imposed by consistency, genre and other factors. Perhaps commercial appeal will also feature in some of my decisions. But these are soft constraints in the sense that I can always choose to override them. There are no hard limits to what I can write about my fictional creations. It is this that rules out the possibility of fiction being true in an external sense of

MY LIFE AS A FICTIONAL CHARACTER

corresponding to a reality that lies outside it. The internal reality of fiction is created entirely by what I write, and I can write whatever I want. But reality – in the external sense that lies outside fiction – cannot simply be whatever I want. Fiction depends entirely on what an author writes, but reality does not. Therefore, at the heart of the so-called falsity of fiction is *dependent existence*: the being of fictional characters is fixed – determined – by what is written of them. Dependent existence is the essence of fiction, and falsity is a consequence of dependent existence. From dependent existence there also follows something that is peculiarly central to the story I am going to tell you in this book. Anything with dependent existence is *incompletable* and, as such, will never, definitively, die.

What did I do on the morning of 24 April 1988? I don't remember, and neither, I am pretty sure, does anyone else. I have my suspicions based on what was going on in my life at the time. I was a few weeks away from submitting my doctoral dissertation at Oxford, and my guess is that I was working on that, likely in my room, in a shared house in Summertown, sitting in my pyjamas – my bed was a few feet away from my desk – writing. Whether or not my guess is correct, I was obviously doing something, even if it was only sleeping in. Moreover, whatever it was that I was doing, it is a fact that I was doing it. There is, as philosophers sometimes put it, a *fact of the matter* about what I was doing, even if no one knows what this fact is. The same is true of any

THE BOOK OF MEMORY

other time since my birth in 1962. At any moment since my emergence into the world, I have always been somewhere doing something, or somewhere having something happen to me. Whatever and wherever this was, it is a fact that I did it or that it happened to me there. At every moment in my life, there corresponds a fact of the matter about what this moment contained. This correspondence of moments and facts will continue to the moment of my death. The same is true of you. Philosophers sometimes put this by saying that we, people who happen to be real, are *ontically fat*.

Coming from the mouths of philosophers, ontically fat is not a bad way to be. Indeed, it denotes a preferred kind of being or way of existing. The term 'ontically' derives from the ancient Greek for being, *ōn*, and means pertaining to the being of something, or the way in which that thing exists. My being, and yours too, is generally thought to be fat. Being ontically fat is not the same thing as being physically fat – although, to be honest, I could stand to lose a few pounds – and is perhaps best understood by contrasting it with someone who is ontically thin.

What did Sherlock Holmes do on the morning of, say, 24 April 1888? What, for example, did he have for breakfast that morning? My acquaintance with Conan Doyle's Sherlock Holmes corpus is not what it might be, but perhaps, in one of his stories, Conan Doyle addressed Holmes's breakfast choices on that morning. Assuming he did not, what can we say about this question and possible answers to it? The most reasonable interpretation is that the question has

MY LIFE AS A FICTIONAL CHARACTER

no answer. If Conan Doyle nowhere addressed Holmes's breakfast elections on this day, there is neither a right nor a wrong answer to this question. We cannot even say that Holmes had nothing for breakfast, for this would imply that Holmes refrained from eating, and there is nothing Conan Doyle wrote which would establish this. There is no fact of the matter about what, if anything, Holmes ate for breakfast on this day. On the other hand, there is a fact of the matter about what I had for breakfast on the same day one hundred years later. There is such a fact – and this fact may simply be 'nothing' – even if no one can remember what it is.

Holmes is ontically thin in the sense that his being or existence is fixed, completely, by what is written about him. The existence of the ontically thin is a dependent one. Where nothing has been written, there are no facts about his being and so no questions we can sensibly ask. There is one crucial consequence of this difference between Holmes and me. My being is *completable* and his is not. While I am still alive, of course, my being is incomplete. New chapters in my life are yet to be written, new facts about me will continue to emerge day in, day out. Long may this glorious incompleteness continue. But there will come a time when my being is complete. When I die, my being becomes solidified and fixed. With my death, my being congeals. No new facts about me can be created, although hitherto unknown or forgotten facts may be unearthed, and new ways of thinking about, or conceptualizing, me may also subsequently emerge, assuming anyone can be bothered to do the requisite conceptualizing.

THE BOOK OF MEMORY

The Hundred Years' War, for example, could not have begun life as the Hundred Years' War. That way of understanding it could only have emerged subsequently, when it dragged on for the required length of time. Nevertheless, what is true of me and what is false are fixed by my death. All that I was and all that I was ever going to be are fixed. Through death, my being is, in this sense, completed.

The same is not true of Holmes. Holmes's being is determined by what is written about him. And this writing, in principle, need never end. That Conan Doyle is the creator of Holmes does not mean Holmes's story cannot be continued by someone else. Others – engaged broadly in the genre of fanfiction – might take the character of Holmes and write new works with him as the protagonist. Indeed, Holmes's now famous catchphrase 'Elementary, my dear Watson!' did not issue from the pen of Conan Doyle but from a play written in the 1890s with Holmes as the central protagonist. Conan Doyle came to hate Holmes – seeing him as a distraction from his long-standing dream of writing serious historical fiction – and wished to do away with him long before his seemingly fatal struggle with his nemesis, Professor Moriarty, on the Reichenbach Falls. So why shouldn't someone else take the character of Holmes and run with it?

This, admittedly, raises some interesting questions. Would this new, fanfiction version of Holmes really be Holmes? I'm not sure the question makes sense: what does 'really' mean here? But I don't see any reason for denying that this

MY LIFE AS A FICTIONAL CHARACTER

newly written character is Holmes. We might take note of the great Greek philosopher Plato in understanding the status of this new Holmes. Plato detested the written word. A spoken idea retains a close connection with its author. It always appears, inevitably, in the same place as its author. But an idea captured in written language, Plato thought, is sent into the world on its own, and must make its own way. Others may twist this idea for their own nefarious purposes. Misrepresentation and exploitation are perennial liabilities for any idea that has become enmeshed in words. In its spoken form, an idea is a beloved and cossetted child. In its written form, the idea is an orphan. A fictional character is, in essence, merely a complex idea. Holmes separated from Conan Doyle is an orphaned Holmes, perhaps. Nevertheless, an orphaned Holmes would still be Holmes in the way that an orphaned child is still a child.

If enough people began writing their own Holmes stories, these would inevitably conflict. One story would have Holmes solving a particular crime on a particular day, whereas another would place him elsewhere solving an entirely different crime. The fanfictioned Holmes – in all his possible incarnations – will inevitably end up doing contradictory things, and how can one and the same person do contradictory things? But there seems to be a straightforward answer available: that's just the way it is with fictional characters. I, ontically rotund as I am, cannot do contradictory things. But ontically svelte fictional characters can and often do. They are slim enough to slip

THE BOOK OF MEMORY

through the chains of contradiction. Suppose, for example, that Conan Doyle, perhaps late in life, wrote a story placing Holmes at a certain place on a certain date solving a particular mystery when, in fact – something Conan Doyle had forgotten – an earlier one of his stories placed Holmes on that date in Surrey solving *The Adventure of the Speckled Band*. Given this continuity error, would we really want to say that this character, issuing from the hand of Conan Doyle, and presented by him as Holmes, is not really Holmes? Contradiction in itself does not rule out both figures qualifying as Holmes.

As ontically thin, the being of fictional characters extends as far – only as far, but nevertheless as far – as what has been written about them. This means that fictional characters are always incomplete. No matter what has been written about them, there is always more that can be written. Every time someone writes something new about Holmes, his being becomes a little more complete; a little more extensive, a little denser. More of his being is filled in. But this process is, in principle, incompletable. There is no limit to what you can write about Holmes. Death does not complete Holmes because death can always be rewritten. *The Final Problem*, published in 1893, sees Holmes fall to his death, along with his nemesis Moriarty, at the Reichenbach Falls in Switzerland. But 1903's *The Adventure of the Empty House* sees him brought back from the dead. According to the 1903 story, Holmes didn't, in fact, fall from the cliffs, but secretly climbed them to safety and subsequently went into hiding

MY LIFE AS A FICTIONAL CHARACTER

for several years. There are, of course, numerous mechanisms that can be used to restart stories that were supposed to have ended (including the 'it was only a dream' scenario used in at least one well-known 1970s TV show, and the recently popular 'multiverse' gambit beloved of the Marvel empire). When you are a fictional character, you are never definitively finished. Additions to your being can always be made. Your being is never complete.

Being a fictional character no doubt has its drawbacks. Being ontically thin means that your existence ultimately hinges on someone else and what they write about you. You have no control over who and what you are. Your being is, in this sense, never truly your own. You are an essentially *dependent* being. Nevertheless, there is one notable advantage. You need never die. Death completes the one who dies. An essentially incompletable being never dies. Death is never definitive for such a being.

The foregoing remarks are an uncontroversial summary of the difference between fictional characters and us, an outline of the differences in the type of being – thin versus fat – had by the fictional and the corporeal respectively. This is a summary – a story of sorts – that pretty much everyone believes. But now I am going to introduce a plot twist. This above summary misses something important. We are, of course, not fictional characters. We are not, in general, ontically thin. Nevertheless, there is a facet of us that is. Even better: it's not just any old facet of us, but one that is peculiarly central to who we are. This facet is *memory*.

Memory, I suggested earlier, is nothing like what we have thought it to be. Now we can grasp, in outline, one of the things I meant by this: like fictional characters, our memories are not completable. Memory is written, but – as I'll explore in this book – every time a memory is recalled it must be rewritten. Every time it is recalled, a memory demands and requires completion; but it can never be completed. The possibility of revision haunts every memory. And the person whose memory it is does not even have to be around to draft those revisions. Our memories make us who we are. But in our memories, also, we most closely approximate fictional beings and are, as such, incompletable. Our memories, therefore, are the closest we will ever get to everlasting life.

Part One

THE BOOK OF MEMORY

There is a book. A magic book. A book of blood and bone, certainly, and jacketed with skin. But much, much more than this. All the experiences you have ever had and ever will have are captured in its pages. The first sentence of this book was written at the moment of your birth, and the book will be written until the moment of your death. And beyond that too.

This is a book of redactions: of immense swathes of black, dominating, dark, and depthless, as far as the eye can see. The sentences of this book are bright islands in an oil-black ocean.

A strange book, indeed. Yet even stranger than this is that every time you read it, every time you look at it, these bright islands in the night will change. You will never catch them changing, but they will. They will change precisely because you read them. It is your reading that changes them.

This is your book. This is the book of you.

1

THE PATH OUT OF THE WOODS

I have a memory. I am lying on the floor of a pine woods, face pointed towards the sky, a jagged slash of open blue, framed in needle green. I am trying very hard to do something. I am trying to make myself forget the way home. This is not because I don't want to go home. What I want to do is *find* my way home. And I can only find my way home if I don't yet *know* my way home. Forgetting my way home would be an improbable triumph of the will in the best of circumstances, and it is hindered by the modest dimensions of the woods in which I find myself. But I will do my best. This was a phase that peaked when I was a ten-year-old boy but never went away. I would try to get lost in the woods. I would try to get lost precisely so I could find my way out again.

The first time I came here on my own – although I was never really on my own as Boots, the dog of my boyhood, a thickset, pale-almost-white Labrador, was always bounding along beside me – I almost did get lost. For a few moments, fierce and sweet, I did not know how to get out of the woods. It was the greatest feeling of my young life. In those brief moments, terror and exhilaration strode hand in hand over the soft and springy orange pine carpet. Then they were gone, as quickly as they had come, replaced by the banality of the familiar. I spent much of my childhood trying to snatch these moments back, to wrest them back from time's dark and nameless avenue. It happened only once again, and by then I had long bidden childhood adieu.

It was a long weekend in Amsterdam with the woman who would become my wife. Our flight was an early one, and we weren't able to check in to our hotel for some hours. The Van Gogh Museum beckoned, but, with a certain inevitability, we instead ended up in a café, sampling some of Amsterdam's attractions. Some hours later, we found ourselves standing on the street faced with a puzzle. We had been to the hotel earlier that day and dropped off our luggage, and it was no more than a few blocks away from the café. However, for reasons you might be able to surmise, finding our way back proved much more difficult than I had anticipated. It was bitterly cold, with a blizzard driving in across the Markermeer. I remember my future wife well that day, piercing blue eyes and blonde hair framed in a white sheepskin hood, like a Viking warrioress of old – but, unfortunately, a rather confused one who kept wandering off into the traffic. Anxiety chirruped insistently. 'You will

THE PATH OUT OF THE WOODS

never find the hotel. You will freeze to death here on the streets of Amsterdam.' And then I saw it again. The path out of the woods that I had last walked as a child. The path of my childhood, the way home that meandered up and out of the woods through the sunlit, cow-parsleyed fields above. I took Emma's hand and followed this path through the woods. Our hotel lay at its end. There were, it goes without saying, no woods and no fields – this was the middle of Amsterdam. But there was a path, I swear it: a shining, sunlit path invisible to all but me.

This has all been a little strange so far. I opened with Sherlock Holmes, segued into dark redactional oceans and bright islands of the night, and then continued on with invisible sunlit paths. I am describing the beginnings of a journey, and no part of this journey is less than strange. Some of it is disorientating, some even vertiginous. Other parts are merely improbable. But all the best journeys are the ones where you start out lost. Only when you are lost can you then be found. 'A philosophical problem,' as the philosopher Ludwig Wittgenstein once said, 'has the form: I don't know my way about.' Don't fight being lost in the woods; embrace it. Draw deep into your lungs the redolence of pine. Immerse yourself in the ambiguous embrace of the lost. The woods – the vast wildwoods of ancient history – were always the place where humans end. The wildwood is death, if you do not know how to get out. But there is always a path out of the woods. You must merely learn to see it.

2

SECOND CHANCES

A child is born because his father was just a little too tired to be as careful as he usually is. Coyness bids me to withhold the identity of this future father-of-the-year, but you can no doubt guess of whom I am talking. He was tired because he had spent the previous two days tiling the downstairs patio in the house in France in which he and future mother – as yet blissfully unaware of the beckoning future – were living at this time. He was tiling the patio because they needed to let the house. They needed to do this because they were moving to Miami. This came about because of a contact the man had made many years before, through a woman he used to date. The woman was a rebound from another. The original woman had dumped him after a disastrous trip that, as college students, they had taken together to India. He would not have dated the rebound – hindsight reveals this to him with confidence – if this had not happened, and the chain would have broken down. But it didn't break down and,

SECOND CHANCES

indeed, stretches deeper into the past. The trip to India was a disaster for several reasons but most obviously because both parties contracted bacillary dysentery roughly four days after they arrived. The incubation period for this form of dysentery is three to four days, which means they probably picked it up on the first day of their trip, presumably when they were eating. They ate in only one place that first day. Thus, a child is conceived because twenty years earlier, someone working in a restaurant in Connaught Circus, New Delhi, didn't adequately wash his or her hands before cooking or serving a biryani. Change any of these things and the chain breaks down. The man does not meet the contact, is not moving to Miami, and does not therefore need to tile his patio. He is not so tired and thus a little more careful during the procreative act. This soon-to-be-conceived child will be mid-range Gen-Z, born in Miami, Florida. But his roots stretch all the way out to northern India and back to a time when, God help us all, the New Romantics were still a thing.

I have identified only a few of the more obvious later links in the chain, but it stretches back to the beginning of time. Break any link and it falls apart. From the broken links, new chains are formed. Different people are dispensed with, and different rebounds found. Different patios are tiled by different people. Different children are born. The soon-to-be-conceived child is a miracle of improbability, as all of us are. You might think that the man tiling the patio could have met the same woman anyway. It is certainly possible, I suppose. But there is more to this child being born than the right people meeting. The right egg and sperm must also meet. There may be, on this occasion, only one of the former in play, but there are six million of the latter little bastards swimming around inside the man. How cosmically unlikely that this very sperm should be the one! A moment or two of delay, a second or two of over-eagerness and – bam! – another swimmer crosses the finish line first and the child never exists. A different sperm yields a different zygote. A different zygote yields a different person – no matter how similar this person would be to the actual child. This is what philosophers call the *necessity of origin*.

Children are a second chance. They wipe the tab clean, making of each father and mother a *tabula rasa*. No matter what inanities we have perpetrated in our lives before our children were born, no matter what idiocies we have inflicted on the world and on ourselves, these were all necessary. Without them the chains of history are broken: different links and chains are formed, and this newborn child, held in his mother's arms, would never have existed. In this sense, our children are our redeemers. They turn our stupidities into our necessities. Unfortunately, our redemption lasts only until the final child is conceived, and then the karmic tab grows anew. Twenty-three months between the first conception and what turned out to be the last. Twenty-three months between my two children. That was the extent of my karmic deliverance.

3

METAPHORS

There is, therefore, no such thing as the beginning of you, only beginnings before beginnings before beginnings, stretching back to the birth of the first light. Nevertheless, one can always find *a* beginning of you. There are as many beginnings as there are times we deem significant. Your birth, in the biological sense, seems as good a place as any to assign the status of *beginning*. At the moment of your birth, a path began. A different beginning necessarily means a different path. The result is – must be – a different person. Different beginnings, different paths, different persons. This, too, is the necessity of origin. Whenever there is a beginning that is in fact yours, then it can be no one else's beginning. Since that moment of your upsurge into the world, you have walked a unitary, unified track through space and time. At every moment, you have always been at some place and at some time. You have never been in more than one place at any one time. But you have been in the same place at many different times. You are the track left in reality by a four-dimensional worm.

THE BOOK OF MEMORY

That's the problem with metaphors – they tend to jump around, often without you realizing it. You see what just happened? A worm is unhappy in the sunlight. It tunnels. Thus, I began with a path (a two-dimensional construction), and then seamlessly switched to a tunnel (a three-dimensional alternative). Metaphors are treacherous. They can hold your thinking tightly in their grip, as a newborn baby might grasp his father's finger tightly seconds after being born – oh yes, I remember that and hope I always will – hold it like a spell, ushering it down certain familiar streets, avenues, and often fruitless cul-de-sacs and no-through roads. That, too, is a metaphor, and using a metaphor to explain the problems with metaphors is self-defeating. But I suspect that, as far as human thought goes, that's all we have.

A metaphor is essentially an invitation: why don't you think of things in this way? Thus – metaphorically – whispers the metaphor softly. Thinking is hard. Thoughts have to be diamond hard to last. And the hardest part of thinking is finding the right metaphor. The right invitation. The right picture. The right way of looking at things. A path? A tunnel? Many years of treading the cul-de-sacs and no-through roads of thought have led me to a different picture. Why don't you think of things in this way? Your life is like an immense scroll, a vast parchment, that is first unrolled at birth and rolls out a little more with every passing day, a sturdy scroll that winds its way through space and time without ever tearing. The world writes on this scroll. And, for us, the words of the world are experiences.

METAPHORS

The world writes on many things. The weathering of a rock is a language written in the rock by time and chemistry. But sometimes, in some cases, the world uses a special, and highly idiosyncratic, language: the language of conscious experience. When you see a bright blue sky above you, or feel warm sand between your toes, or smell the salt wind, and hear the ocean's gentle susurration, these experiences are all ways in which the world writes itself upon you. There are more unpleasant ways too, of course. But pleasant or painful, positive or negative, for us and for conscious animals like us, experience is the first language of the world.

Experiences come and are quickly gone, like words written in the sand before an incoming tide. *Einmal ist keinmal*, as an old German proverb says. Once is never. Once is not at all. Once counts for nothing. Experiences are inconsequential unless they are retained. With consciousness, therefore, comes memory. If experiences are the words the world has inscribed on and in us, then memory is the ability to read these words. When you remember, you read what the world has done to you. You read what the world has written in you.

Now imagine the final stage in the construction of you. The scroll, a little arbitrarily I admit, is divided up into twenty-four-hour segments, marked by perforations that allow you to detach one segment from the next. And suppose that at the end of each day, this is precisely what happens. A new segment is detached and is placed, face up, under the previous segments. The result of these collated pages is a book, rather than a scroll. This is the book of you. After

THE BOOK OF MEMORY

your death, this book would be all that is left of you, a record of the experiences the world has written on you between your dawn and your demise. But while you are alive, things are very different. The book is something to which you can return at any time, and as many times as you wish, dipping into the pages as you choose. This is what memory does for you. Memory is the ability to read the book of you. You are, therefore, both the book and the one who reads the book. You are the reader and the read. You are the remembering and the remembered.

4

KINDS OF REMEMBERING

The concept of memory is an exceptionally broad one, encompassing a variety of different things. I remember *how* to tie my shoelaces, ride a bicycle and play the piano. These are examples of *procedural* memory: memory of how to do things. The book of you is not a book of procedural memories. Many different people can tie their shoes, ride their bicycles and play their pianos. Admittedly, as the skill set expands, the number of people who have it diminishes. But it is always possible that two different people can possess precisely the same skills. If the book of you were simply a book of procedural memories, the book of you could, just as easily, also be the book of someone else. The book would not, therefore, be specific to you. Its pages would not describe the person that you, unambiguously, are – you as opposed to an identically skilled someone else.

I remember *that* Paris is the capital of France, that Vesuvius erupted in AD 79 and that the platypus is a monotreme. These

THE BOOK OF MEMORY

are examples of *semantic* memory. Semantic memory is memory of facts. While it may contain them, the book of you is not, essentially, a book of semantic memories. Such memories are not what is distinctive about the book. Semantic memories are beliefs. To say that I remember that Paris is the capital of France, that Vesuvius erupted in AD 79 and that the platypus is a monotreme is equivalent to saying that I believe these things. Not all beliefs are semantic memories – I can have beliefs about the future, for example – but all semantic memories are beliefs. Semantic memories may find their way into the book of you from time to time, but it is always possible – unlikely, but nevertheless possible – that two different people could have precisely the same semantic memories. You and I might both remember that Paris is the capital of France, that Vesuvius erupted in AD 79 and that the platypus is a monotreme. And it might be that for every fact you know, I know the same fact, and vice versa. Unlikely, as I say, but possible.

It is true that some facts – and, therefore, some semantic memories – are *autobiographical*. I remember that I was born in Newport. But someone else might have that autobiographical memory too: he remembers that he was born in Newport. I remember that I am Mark Rowlands. But it is possible that he shares my name. Perhaps I was born in St Joseph's, while he was born in the Royal Gwent Hospital. This differential fact would distinguish us, but only if we remember it, and it may be that we have both forgotten the hospitals of our birth. While there are autobiographical facts

KINDS OF REMEMBERING

that distinguish us, it might be – unlikely but possible – that you and I have both forgotten all those distinguishing facts. In short, if the book of you were a book of semantic memories – memories of facts – it would be possible that the book of you is also the book of someone else. It is this possibility that is crucial, and not its likelihood. It is not possible for you to be someone else. If it is possible for a book of semantic memories to be equally applicable to someone else – if there is nothing that makes it, essentially, the book of you as opposed to the book of another – then this book would not capture you. It would not capture the essence of the person you are.

The book of you, therefore, is not a book of skills and it is not a book of remembered facts. It is a book of experiences, for your experiences are yours and yours alone. Experiences are recalled in a specific type of memory, known as *episodic* memory. The book of you is, fundamentally, a book of such memories. The memory of lying in a pine woods, looking at the sky, and trying to will myself to forget the way home is an episodic memory. I don't merely remember *that* I used to do this. I remember doing it. If procedural memory is remembering *how*, and semantic memory is remembering *that*, then episodic memory is simply remembering.

I remember that Vesuvius erupted in AD 79 – a semantic memory – but I don't remember it erupting. If I did, that would be an episodic memory. The eruption of Vesuvius was, admittedly, an episode or event, but remembering that this episode occurred is not enough to make the memory episodic. Suppose, however, that I had a time machine – episodic memory is sometimes described as *mental time travel* – and could travel back to Pompeii on the fateful day of the eruption. In such circumstances, I might later remember the thunderous noise of the eruption and the sight of the vast cloud of smoke and ash filling the sky from horizon to horizon. I might remember seeing the ash beginning to descend on the city, smelling the stench of sulphur in the air. If these experiential details were in place, then I would now remember the episode of Vesuvius erupting *as* an episode I had formerly experienced. That is what these experiential details do: collectively they present an episode to me *as* one that I have formerly witnessed. This remembering of an episode *as* one I have formerly experienced is the essence of episodic memory. The experiential details that allow one to remember an episode in this way are sometimes referred to as the *episodicity* of the memory.

Their episodicity means that episodic memories differ from other kinds of memory in at least one crucial way: I am *in* my episodic memories in a way I can never be in their procedural and semantic counterparts. This is why my book of episodic memories is specific to me – and why your book would be specific to you – in a way that a book of procedural memories or semantic memories could never be. When, courtesy of the time machine, I experienced the sounds and sights and smells of Vesuvius erupting – the thunderous noise, the vast ash cloud, the stench of sulphur – these put me in my memory in the sense that these are things

KINDS OF REMEMBERING

I remember having experienced. The noise is a noise that *I* heard, the ash cloud one that *I* saw, the sulphur stench one that *I* smelled. That's how I remember it. Before I travelled back in time, I had merely a semantic memory of the eruption of Vesuvius. Having the experiences, on the other hand, would afford me an episodic memory of this event. And it did so by, in effect, placing me in the memory. This is not in the sense that the memory is about me. The memory is still about the eruption of Vesuvius. Rather, I am in the memory in the sense that the eruption is now presented *as* one that *I* formerly experienced. For a memory of mine to qualify as episodic, there needs to be an episode, I need to experience it, and I need to remember it *as* an episode *I* formerly experienced.

This presence of the person in their episodic memories – the defining feature of episodic memory – is sometimes called *autonoesis*. The book of you is a book of autonoesis. It is a book made up of episodic memories in which the events of your life are portrayed, precisely, as ones that you did or ones that happened to you.

5

HIGHLY SUPERIOR AND SEVERELY DEFICIENT

At this point, the old academic in me – he's still there, unfortunately, scratching away at ideas – feels compelled to chime in with some notes on the nuances of the distinction between episodic and semantic memory. As usual, he will only complicate matters, but I shall indulge him this once. You can safely skip to the next section if you like. Consider, this academic requests, the case of R.B. As a result of neurological damage incurred in a car accident, R.B. suffered a loss, or at least severe attenuation, of his sense of what he described as his 'ownership' of memories of events that occurred before the accident. In his words:

> What I realized was that I did not 'own' any memories that came before my injury. I knew things that came before my injury. In fact, it seemed that my memory was

HIGHLY SUPERIOR AND SEVERELY DEFICIENT

just fine for things that happened going back years in the past ... I could answer any question about where I lived at different times in my life, who my friends were, where I went to school, activities I enjoyed, etc. But none of it was 'me'. It was the same sort of knowledge I might have about how my parents met or the history of the Civil War or something like that.

R.B.'s condition is sometimes known as *severely deficient autobiographical memory*, or SDAM. The label is misleading. Some of your memories are about you, and some are not. The former are known as *autobiographical* memories. Autobiographical memories can be episodic – I might vividly remember, for example, the arrival of my family's first colour TV – a rental from Rediffusion – one Saturday lunchtime when I was (roughly) eight years old, and a subsequent afternoon spent in technicolour glory, watching things I would never have bothered to watch on the old black and white. This is an episodic memory and also an autobiographical one. Indeed, arguably, all episodic memories are autobiographical because the person who remembers is, in the sense I have already explained with the example of Mount Vesuvius, always in them. Episodic memories are autonoetic, and therefore, in one clear sense, autobiographical. But not all autobiographical memories need be episodic. I remember that I was born in Newport. But I have no episodic memory of being born there. This memory is autobiographical – it is about me – but also semantic. The expression *severely deficient autobiographical memory* is misleading, at least as a label for R.B.'s condition, because his semantic autobiographical memories are just fine. It's just that these are all he has. His episodic memories have gone because he no longer has the kind of experiences required for him to remember episodes *as* ones he formerly experienced. R.B. knows intellectually that certain events happened in his past – happened to him. But he does not experience them as such. R.B.'s condition would better be labelled SDEM: severely deficient *episodic* memory.

R.B., you might be happy to learn, later recovered. His episodic memories slowly returned. Until recently, the received wisdom was that cases such as R.B.'s are extremely rare and restricted to people with neurological damage. However, more recent studies have suggested that this kind of deficiency of episodic memory might be far more widespread and present in otherwise neurologically healthy people. Like R.B., such people are unable to vividly recollect personal past episodes as ones that formerly happened to them. That is, they do not remember such episodes as ones they formerly experienced although, like R.B., they can usually infer that such episodes once happened to them. Unlike R.B., for them there is no obvious neurological damage that would explain this inability. Therefore, rather than being an isolated phenomenon, restricted to those with certain sorts of neurological damage, it is likely that SDAM is quite widely distributed in the general population. It exists not as an all-or-nothing phenomenon, but as one that comes in

HIGHLY SUPERIOR AND SEVERELY DEFICIENT

degrees. It's not as if you either have SDAM or you don't; rather, it's that many people have some degree of SDAM. Rather than being a disorder, SDAM is better thought of as a certain range on a spectrum, with only the outer limit of this range being linked to pathology.

At the opposite end of the spectrum from SDAM, we find HSAM: *highly superior autobiographical memory*. For reasons evinced in the paragraph before last, it is probably more accurately dubbed HSEM – highly superior episodic memory. People with HSAM not only recall past episodes with an incredible level of detail, they also tend to retain far more episodes than the average person. HSAM also is not so much a point on a spectrum but a range. At the extreme end of the HSAM range is *hyperthymesia*: the inability to forget anything. Your episodic memory can be more or less highly superior or more or less severely deficient. More likely, if you are statistically normal, it will be somewhere in between – in the comfortable middle range of the superior–deficient spectrum.

The book of you is a book of episodic memories. But that is only a rough approximation of a more complex reality. Instead of thinking of memories as either episodic or not, think instead in terms of *degrees of episodicity*. My memory of the arrival of the Rowlands family's first colour TV is richly episodic because it contains the kind of experiential details that allow me to remember this episode as one I have experienced before. Without these details, I might have merely a semantic memory of this event: I would remember simply that my first colour TV arrived when I was (roughly) eight years old – as I might remember that I was born in Newport. But suppose, the ravages of time being what they are, these experiential details are slowly denuded. With this gradual stripping away of experiential details the memory becomes progressively less episodic and more semantic in character. In other words, instead of thinking of the distinction between episodic and semantic as a dichotomy, we should think of it as a spectrum – a spectrum of varying degrees of episodicity. Once we get sufficiently far enough over to the deficient end of the spectrum – as we would, for example, in the case of R.B. – we might no longer be inclined to regard what remains as an episodic memory at all, but only as the semantic remnant of such a memory.

We are all different – the episodicity of our memories varies from one person to another and, indeed, from one memory to another. It is better to think of the book of you as a book not of episodic memories, but of memories of varying degrees of episodicity.

6

THE BOOK OF YOU

To describe you as a book of memories does, admittedly, sound a little strange. But try it out: I think it will grow on you. You don't look like a book, of course, but that's superficial. Books come in many forms. And you've no doubt heard that you should never judge a book by its cover. Your cover is skin rather than card or cloth. The words that make you up may not look like words, but they are. They are words written in neural ink, the electrochemical contours and configurations, eddies and ensembles inscribed in the brain. Every thought, every feeling, every emotion and every experience you have ever had will have taken the form of this neural writing. Words inked into a page, or words burned into neural architecture: *we are all just words somewhere.*

Books, of course, are not only books of words. There are books of images: photographs, drawings, paintings. There are also joke books, and children's books, where you open a page and some combination of sounds — a song, a chorus of farmyard animals, perhaps – is emitted. The book of you might be like an e-book, a book of pixels. Or hypertext: you click on a link, and a scene from the past is replayed for you, on your own personal YouTube channel. You click on another link, and the smell of newly cut grass on an early summer's day, the first cut of the summer, just after the chill of spring has left the air, insinuates its way into your nostrils. Scenes, sounds, scents are all found in the book of you. Whether a memory is a word, a picture, a video, a scent, a sound, a taste or a feeling matters not at all to me. What I want to insist on is that whatever memories are, you are a book of them.

The genre of this book is, of course, autobiography. This is a metaphor, and I choose it because whatever else is true of an autobiography, it is – or is supposed to be – a record of the past. Embodied in any autobiography is a recognition of the predominance of the past over the present and the future. There is much more than memory that goes into a human life – this is too obvious to require repeating. There are thoughts, feelings, hopes, fears. There are beliefs, deeply held or otherwise. There are desires, mundane or troubling. There are dreams for a future that is not yet but might come to be. But memory, nevertheless, has a peculiar centrality to each one of us.

The belief in the predominance of the past is grounded in the thought with which this book opened: what could make you the person you are, on this path through space and time that is your life, other than the things you have done and the things that have happened to you? And how could these things that were done and happened be retained if not through memory? 'Poor creatures that we are, our life is so vain that it is nothing but a reflection of our memories,' as Chateaubriand once put it. The *now* is of dubious reality. There is little of substance to it. It exists as an imaginary and always shifting point constructed from memories of the past and anticipations of the future. The *now*, therefore, cannot make you what you are. Neither, it seems, can the future: merely a promise or possibility and as such entirely diaphanous. With the past, however, there is the solidity of the having been. The past is written, or so we think. It is, accordingly, your past that makes you who you are, and your past is retained only in memories. If you were a book, therefore, you would be a book of memories.

You might not want to give up on the future quite so easily. Insubstantial it may be, but it is still true that we live much of our lives in futures that may or may not ever become real. Think of everything you do today so that a certain tomorrow, and not others, might be born. It has been so for much of your life. We are, in this sense, *beings-towards-a-future*, as Martin Heidegger once put it. This is true. But Heidegger also acknowledged that our being-towards-a-future is decisively shaped by our *already-being-in-the-world*. Your desire for a future of a certain sort, shape or character, a desire in which you may invest decades of labour, is a desire that has been inscribed in you by the past. Nevertheless, regarding the more general point, there is nothing in the metaphor of the book of memory that is anathema to a future yet to be built. This future exists only in the imagination, of course. But memory and imagination cannot be separated.

Imagination is built into the book of you because in life, imagination and memory are two facets of one and the same thing. Recall: you are both writer and reader of the book of memories. You write memories when you go out into the world and have experiences. You remember when you read back what has been written. But imagination is part of what it is to read. Reading is never simply a matter of looking at words and understanding their meaning. You must also understand their *significance*. Suppose that in a novel a certain event occurs – the plan of the protagonist unravels, for example – and the event carries within itself future possibilities or probabilities. What is going to happen now? What does this mean for so-and-so? Disaster beckons, perhaps. But is it avoidable? Or is it inevitable? It is not bare events that you encounter in a novel but events laden with significance. This significance is a matter of their implications. And we understand these implications through imagination.

The same is true of a biography or autobiography. Let us suppose you are reading an autobiography. You know very little about the person who is the subject of this book. In particular, you don't know how his life ultimately turns out – just as you don't know how your life is ultimately going to turn out. As events in this person's life unfold before your eyes on the pages of the book, you will, if you are remotely engaged in this person's story, not merely record what is happening but try to understand its significance. And you do this by imagining what these events will mean for the person and the future course of his life.

The book of you is nothing if not an autobiography – one written by you and for your eyes only – and, as such, the same general points apply. You don't just remember bare events from your life; what you remember is laden with, permeated by, significance – sometimes great, sometimes small (insignificance is just another form, a limiting case, of significance). Sometimes the significance of an event has already shown itself, played out its part on the stage of your life. But sometimes the significance of past events has yet to become clear. What will they mean for you and your life? You don't yet know. For such events – those you remember but whose ramifications are less than clear – you try to ascertain their significance through anticipation, and thereby through imagination. When what you remember has significance as yet undisclosed – and it is perhaps rare for the significance of a remembered event to ever be fully disclosed – to remember is, at the same time, to imagine. The connection between memory and imagination is deep and unbreakable. To remember is to imagine, and to imagine is to remember. Through memory you can imagine your future. And through imagination you can remember your past. A book of memories is also a book of imagination. Things couldn't be any other way.

Part Two

THE WATERS OF LETHE

In Greek mythology, Lethe is a river, the river of forgetfulness, and the last stage in the journey to the underworld, before you enter the Elysian Fields, if that is your destination. Lethe receives the wretched and desolate, the exhausted and broken, and carries them to the other side, not restored – for who they were is gone – but whole again and happy. The Greeks understood well that forgetting is a precondition of paradise.

But I recommend to you a rather different picture of Lethe. Think of Lethe not as a river but as an ocean, one already dark and stretching towards a yet darker horizon. The book of you is dominated by night-black seas, sprinkled with shining-island sentences: tiny islets of remembrance, glimmering in the night. But neither the ocean nor the islands are what they seem to be.

The currents here are treacherous. And the sands are always subtly shifting.

7

PATRICK

My sons' maternal great-grandfather, Patrick, died of a heart attack. This was, in the circumstances, a merciful end. Before it happened, he had developed Alzheimer's. Every time I saw him, his decline was unmistakable. Before too long, he was none too sure of the identity of even the closest members of his family. Then temporal confusion set in and Patrick became lost in time. An accomplished escape artist, Patrick would sometimes disappear, apparently wandering the highways and byways of his youth, not able to find his way home, not realizing that he was a man of more than seventy years and being horrified when reality impinged on his illusions. Nevertheless, I could never quite shake the feeling that, despite the catastrophic memory loss and frequent brushes with bewilderment, there was always something about him – something there – that was recognizably Patrick. In catastrophic memory loss of this sort, what remains can sometimes shine through what is lost.

Patrick had little formal education. He spent quite a bit of his adult life working in the shipyards of the UK and became

THE BOOK OF MEMORY

an accomplished welder. But reading was his passion: reading and telling people about what he had been reading. He was a fount of interesting stories. Some were about his life. Others were about the things he had read in books. Towards the end they were sometimes, perhaps, a mixture of the two – but none the worse for that. The stories stayed with Patrick, even when much else had departed, even when he couldn't remember who his wife, daughters or granddaughters were. The stories were still there; indeed, in some ways they were enhanced. I gather that's how it is sometimes with those in the grip of dementia. Newer memories are quickly lost, but the older ones, from a lifetime ago, can still be there, shining and pristine. It is as if some memories can only be found when others have been peeled away: as if memories are arranged like the layers of an onion. These memories that are found are, in some ways, like new. But they are also unmoored, drifting, lost in time. There is no longer enough land left surrounding for them to have a place in a person's life.

In the end, I think that what remained of Patrick was not so much a story, but a *style*. The story had broken down: too much had been eroded by the waters of Lethe. But there remained an *existential* style: a certain way of being. This style was perfectly visible. I can picture him, the last time I saw him, sitting in the pub, a pint of Murphy's in his hand, quietly and engagingly telling a story. It is entirely appropriate that I have forgotten what this story was about, because that was what was happening to Patrick. It is the quiet sitting, the gentle voice, the understated erudition: that is what was significant. This is the sort of thing I have in mind when I talk of Patrick's existential style. We all have an existential style.

The book of memory is an uncanny book. Its most noticeable feature, unless you have hyperthymesic recall, is the vast sea of black — the dark ink of redaction — that dominates almost every page. We have, the vast majority of us, forgotten far more than we remember. This is true even of those yet in the first bloom of youth, whose minds are steel memory traps compared with my old, rusty-and-far-from-trusty sieve. We tend to think of catastrophic memory loss as reserved for those like Patrick, those with degenerative brain conditions. But this is not so. Most of us suffer from it, and all of us will eventually. How could these vast swathes of redactions, dominating almost every page, represent anything less than memory loss of catastrophic proportions?

Lethe is an ocean, dark and vast. The islands of remembrance are comparatively small, sparse and scattered. That so much of the book of you is dominated by redaction creates a deep puzzle, perhaps as deep as the ocean itself. Your memories are supposed to make you who you are. It is the things you have done and the things that have happened to you that make you who you are, and memory is the most obvious, if not the only, record of these things past. But it is such a scanty record, capturing only a tiny fraction of your past. How can your memories make you who you are if almost all of the things that memory is supposed to record — the things you have done and the things that have happened to you — have been forgotten?

8

RILKEAN MEMORIES

The *content* of a memory is what that memory is about – what it is a memory *of*. Catastrophic memory loss is, thus, a loss of the contents of memories. The contents of a person's memories disappear – as they did in the case of Patrick. But style can survive the loss of much content. It can survive those vast night-black swathes of content lost – precisely because, sometimes, perhaps more often than we recognize, the content that is lost returns precisely in the form of style.

Once upon a time, one of my sons asked me a very good question. Working our way around Europe, we'd spent the last few days in Paris, and I was talking about all the great memories that we were going to have from the trip once it was over. Some non-immediate family members had speculated that my sons were too young to remember anything of the trip, an opinion this particular son had overheard. His question was: *Where do our memories go when we lose them?* Often, when we lose something, it is because it is somewhere

RILKEAN MEMORIES

else. My iPhone is in the car while I am in the house looking for it. The delinquent item doesn't actually have to be anywhere else though. Not so long ago, I spent at least ten minutes looking for a baseball cap that I subsequently discovered was on my head. Still, the general idea is that some things are lost because they are not where we are looking for them. Other things, on the other hand, are lost because they are nowhere at all: they no longer exist – youth, beauty, dreams, and *les neiges d'antan*. So, the question is: are lost memories like the first sort of lost thing (misplaced) or the second (gone for good)?

The standard view is that they are like the second: when memories are lost, it is because they no longer exist. But the first option has attracted some adherents. Freud, perhaps, travelled some distance in this direction, arguing that memories of malign episodes from one's past could live on even after they have seemingly disappeared, exerting a baleful influence on a subject's psyche in the present. But Freud, one should remember, talked mainly of repressed *desires* rather than memories. And even if we understand his claim as referring to memory, it is far from the idea that any apparently forgotten memory can live on in this way. Freud's concern was only with a (hopefully small) subset of memories, malign ones, protection from which required the intervention of psychic defence mechanisms.

A more uncompromising position is taken by the poet Samuel Taylor Coleridge, who at least flirted with the idea that no memory was ever really lost in the second sense: 'For

THE BOOK OF MEMORY

what is forgetfulness? Renew the state of affection or bodily feeling, same or similar – sometimes dimly similar – and instantly the trains of forgotten thought rise up from their living catacombs.' Proust seemed to think something similar, as did the French philosopher Henri Bergson. I think there is much truth to this idea, although not in the way Coleridge thought.

Not only was my son's question a very good one, it was also asked at a very good time. If he hadn't asked it, I might not have been suitably attuned to the following passage, which I happened to be reading on that trip around Europe. The passage is from *The Notebooks of Malte Laurids Brigge*, written by Rainer Maria Rilke, and the Bohemian poet's only excursion into the art form of the novel. I must admit, I have a curious obsession with this book. I don't think it is a great novel. But I do think the first twenty or thirty pages are great. In fact, if anyone has written something better, I'm unacquainted with it. It all falls apart, dramatically, after that – but that's hardly unexpected: Rilke was, after all, a poet, not a novelist. I say all this with a view to explaining, if not excusing, the gratuitous length of the following quotation: I'm afraid I simply can't help myself. The relevant part is in italics – and these are mine, not Rilke's:

> To write a single verse, one must see many cities, and men and things; one must get to know animals and the flight of birds, and the gestures that the little flowers make when they open out to the morning. One must be able to return

RILKEAN MEMORIES

in thought to roads in unknown regions, to unexpected encounters, and to partings that had been long foreseen ... There must be memories of many nights of love, each one unlike the others, of the screams of women in labour, and of women in childbed, light and blanched and sleeping, shutting themselves in. But one must also have been beside the dying, must have sat beside the dead in a room with open windows and with fitful noises. *And still it is not yet enough to have memories. One must be able to forget them when they are many and one must have the immense patience to wait until they come again. For it is the memories themselves that matter. Only when they have turned to blood within us, to glance and gesture, nameless and no longer to be distinguished from ourselves – only then can it happen that in a most rare hour the first word of a poem arises in their midst and goes forth from them.*

Rilke is talking about the importance of memory – or, more precisely, of a certain kind of transformation that memory might undergo – for artistic (specifically poetic) creation. But I think his idea has much broader significance.

The general contours of the transformation Rilke had in mind are clear. We begin with episodic memories of relatively familiar sorts. Some of these memories are of *specific* episodes: of encounters, partings, of women screaming in childbirth, of the noises in the room where you sat next to your dead father. Some are more *general*: the gesture that small flowers make when they open in the morning. And others seem to be a curious mixture of the particular and the general: many nights of love, each one different from all the others. Next, the memory fades and eventually disappears: 'one must be able to forget them'. But the memory lives on and can later return in another, very different, form. The memory has become 'blood', 'glance and gesture', 'nameless and no longer to be distinguished' from the person whose memory it was.

We can explain this process in terms of a distinction between the *act* of remembering and the *content* of memory. The content of memory – what the memory is about – is lost, but the act of remembering lives on. It cannot, however, live on as an act of remembering for there is, now, nothing remembered in this act. Therefore, it lives on in a new form: blood, glance and gesture, nameless. The culmination of this transformative process we might label *Rilkean memories*. It doesn't really matter whether we think of these Rilkean items as memories or as things that memories have become, things into which memories have mutated – Rilkean post-memories, as we might then call them. Indeed, so little do I care about whether these are really memories, that I'm as happy to talk of *Rilkean forgetting* as of Rilkean memory. Either way, a Rilkean memory, or post-memory, or forgetting, carries a trace of your past within it, and so links you to that past. The past lives on in you not as memories in the familiar sense but, rather, as their Rilkean counterparts.

9

A WAKE-UP CALL ON WIMBLEDON COMMON

Paris – where my son's decisive question was asked – was part of a larger trip. I was in Europe for six months, with my wife and children, and Hugo, our German Shepherd. A book of mine had come out earlier that year, *Running with the Pack*, ostensibly about running, but really about answering the question of the meaning of life. For the record, I thought I nailed that answer, in a little over 200 pages to boot. But no one seemed to notice that the book was about the meaning of life, and most of the criticisms of the book were that it didn't explain how to run faster. Serves me right for trying to be subtle. I came up with a better answer later, anyway. To the meaning of life, that is. How to run faster is a much harder problem.

In the interests of shifting a few copies, my publishers had me doing all sorts of ill-advised things. One day, in collaboration with London's School of Life (yes, that's a thing), they had arranged for me to do a running seminar on Wimbledon Common in southwest London with interested, and paying, members of the general public. I took our dog Hugo along with me. A bit of us running, a bit of me talking, a bit of eating, that sort of thing. The running part was a major embarrassment, as it turned out I was, by some distance (literally), the worst runner there. I suspect even Hugo might have been a bit embarrassed by me. Any illusions I might have harboured that I was a halfway decent runner died on the common that day.

There was, nevertheless, a highly instructive segment of the day that involved a seminar with a running coach, and I was able to ask him about a little problem I'd been having with my calves, which seemed to me to tear far more often than they really should. Indeed, part of the reason I wasn't in shape for the Wimbledon debacle was because of a calf tear I had picked up a few weeks before while in France, running in the distinctly hilly terrain of Lyon. The coach took a quick look at my running form and said my calf problem was because I wasn't lifting my knees high enough. If I did that, more strain would be taken by the quads and hamstrings which, being bigger muscles than the calves, were better able to handle it. Challenge accepted. I worked and worked on correcting my form, and a few weeks later, it was sorted. What happened next, do you think?

Knee pain, distinctly unpleasant knee pain, that's what. And then I remembered: I used to have this problem years

A WAKE-UP CALL ON WIMBLEDON COMMON

ago, and then it just went away. Now I understood. My idiosyncratically low knee lift was probably an unconscious, or at least an unwitting, attempt to mitigate my knee issues. Painful experiences, retained in the form of episodic memories, became slightly less painful with suitable adjustments to my gait. My form, therefore, changed incrementally as the result of feedback on the relationship between gait and pain, both during and after my runs, as, over time, I subliminally selected a gait that minimized the unpleasantness.

If things happened in the way I have just described – it is, of course, speculation on my part, but if things did, in fact, happen in this way – then this would be an example of Rilkean memory. Specifically, it is what we can call an *embodied* Rilkean memory: a memory – or, in this case, a series of memories – has become transformed into a bodily tendency to run in a certain idiosyncratic, but knee-protecting, way. An embodied Rilkean memory exists when the content of a memory is lost but the act of remembering lives on as a bodily habit, tendency or disposition. This running style – 'blood, glance and gesture', as Rilke described it – is what my former memories have become, what they have turned into, through a process of (Rilkean) mutation.

For someone in this situation, someone with a Rilkean memory, there are two possibilities. The first is that, like me, the former memories come flooding back. 'Oh, now I understand! I must have been running in such a way to compensate for those knee issues I now remember I had.' But this may not happen. I might never have recalled my previous unpleasant knee pain, and so might never have really understood why my running took on this peculiar form. In both scenarios I have a Rilkean memory. But in the second scenario, the Rilkean memory is *all* that remains of my former memories. The Rilkean memory would now be my only connection to this aspect of my past.

In his book *The Poetics of Space*, Gaston Bachelard, a French philosopher of the first half of the twentieth century, provides a nice example of what I am calling embodied Rilkean memory. The house we were born in, he argues, is physically inscribed in us as a group of 'organic habits'. Even after many years away, upon our return we find ourselves adjusting to the idiosyncrasies of the house. We would 'not stumble on the rather high step', and we 'push the door that creaks with the same gesture'. Let's suppose that, as a teenager, I used to engage in habitual surreptitious nocturnal activities, such as returning to the house much later than I was supposed to. If I did, then it would be important that I did not stumble on a high step or allow the door to emit loud creaks. Upon my return to this house many years later, I, once again, might not stumble on that very high step, but not because I remember, in the standard sense, the step being high. Rather, as I reach the step, I just find myself increasing the size of my stride. The memory has become an 'organic habit' – the tendency to behave in this way when I reach the step. I open the door in a certain way – one that minimizes its creaking – not because I remember that it creaked, but because a pattern of behaviour has become inscribed in my

A WAKE-UP CALL ON WIMBLEDON COMMON

body and my neural infrastructure. This pattern, however, is activated only in the presence of this specific door. These tendencies have insinuated their way into my behaviour through repetition and necessity. Philosophers call these behavioural tendencies *dispositions*, and they are examples of embodied Rilkean memories. Standard memories of the step and the door might have been lost – I have no episodic recollection of either – but their Rilkean counterparts live on. The form these memories of home have now assumed is Rilkean and embodied.

10

HOME, AGAIN

A couple of weeks after my encounter with the running coach, when my ill-fated attempt to change my running technique had yet to reach its painful denouement, we were staying near Hay-on-Wye – a town straddling the Wales–England border, and roughly thirty miles from where I had grown up. I was speaking at the Hay Festival on the topic of, you've guessed it, memory. In fact, it was there that the idea of Rilkean memory started to crystallize in my sluggish mind. This had a lot to do with a run I took one morning with Hugo along the banks of the river Wye, through fields of friendly, inquisitive cows. Hugo was five years old at the time, and in his pomp. There was something strange about this run, something about it that felt very, very right, as if this was how things were supposed to be. This feeling of rightness, of properness, puzzled me. My runs didn't usually feel like that, I assure you. I was in my fifties now, and my runs were slowly but discernibly turning into slogs. This

HOME, AGAIN

run was anything but that. It's true, this was the honeymoon period for my legs, after I'd changed my running technique long enough to feel the improvement in my calves, but before my knees started realizing they'd been here and done this before. But I don't think that was the explanation for this uncanny feeling of rightness, at least certainly not the whole story. Then it hit me. This is how it would have been when I was a boy! A river on one side of me, a steep hillside on the other, and a dog running next to me, matching his stride to mine. Different river, different hillside and different dog, but the overall *gestalt* was the same. I have few standard memories of those days of my youth: flashes, fragments of memories at most. If I am right in these speculations, my memories of those times live on in a new form: they live on as a certain kind of mood – emotion – that assails me when the present and this happy past most closely align. In these moments of alignment, the veil between the present and the past is, perhaps, at its thinnest, and I can see, dimly, uncertainly, what I once was and will never be again, running through these fields of memory turned golden by the morning sun.

If this explanation is correct – and, as in the case of embodied Rilkean memory, I have to accept that it is only a theory – then what I have just described to you is what we might call an *affective* Rilkean memory. Affective Rilkean memories are feelings, emotions, moods, and states of that ilk. Like embodied Rilkean memories, these affective counterparts are the remains, the remnants, of former memories.

THE BOOK OF MEMORY

Sometimes they are all that remain of those memories. But a trace of the past lives on in these affective Rilkean memories. They bind me to my past as deeply as, and perhaps more deeply than, any standard memory ever could.

There is a useful fictional example of what is, in effect, an affective Rilkean memory, courtesy of a book I read to my sons on that book-promoting, question-asking, coach-consulting, knee-shredding trip around Europe. If my sons had never existed, I might at this point be talking about Proust, his tea and his madeleine cake. But at that time they left me scant time to read things like *À la recherche*. On the other hand, they encouraged my reading of certain other works, including, among others, *The Wind in the Willows* (although I have to admit their enthusiasm for this classic was always somewhat tepid). Here is a passage from that book that captures very nicely what I have in mind by affective Rilkean memory. The passage discusses a strange feeling that one day affects Mole:

> We others who have long lost the more subtle of the physical senses have not even the proper terms to express an animal's intercommunication with his surroundings, living or otherwise, and have only the word 'smell', for instance, to include the whole range of delicate thrills which murmur in the nose of the animal night and day, summoning, warning, inciting, repelling. It was one of those mysterious fairy calls from out of the void that suddenly reached Mole in the darkness, making him

HOME, AGAIN

tingle through and through with its very familiar appeal, while as yet he could not clearly remember what it was. He stopped dead in his tracks, his nose searching hither and thither in its efforts to recover the fine filament, the telegraphic current that had so strongly moved him. A moment and he had caught it again; and with it this time came recollection in its fullest flood. Home! That is what they meant, those caressing appeals, those soft touches wafted through the air, those invisible little hands pulling and tugging, all one way.

Mole is the subject of certain sensations or feelings: of a 'telegraphic current', of 'caressing appeals', of 'soft touches' and 'invisible little hands pulling and tugging, all one way'. These are examples of affective Rilkean memories. In their purest form, affective Rilkean memories consist in sensations, feelings and moods that have arisen through the degeneration of run-of-the-mill episodic memories. The content of these memories has become lost, and what remains – or has taken its place – is an affective Rilkean memory. These are what Mole's memories of home have become: the affective Rilkean form they have now assumed. Prior to the onset of 'recollection in its fullest flood' – and on another day, this recollection might never have occurred – when Mole realizes where he is and what these feelings mean, these are all that remain of Mole's memories of home.

11

THE RIVERBANK

A book is always more than its content. It is also its style. A book is not simply what it says, it is also the way it says it. A book of memories is no more a mere collection of memories than an ordinary book is just a collection of sentences. The sentences must be organized in the right way. And for each sentence we can ask two different questions: 'What does the sentence say?' and 'How does it say it?' The way in which sentences of a book are organized and the way in which they say what they say are two components of the *style* of a book.

Imagine this. A discovery has been made of thousands of pages of what appear to be fiction. They appear to be fiction because they – sometimes charmingly, sometimes alarmingly – detail the lives of certain creatures that live on a riverbank. There is a mole, a rat, a toad and a badger, and many other creatures too. However, these pages were discovered in a shattered basement, strewn all over the floor. Many of the pages are utterly illegible due to water damage and other misfortunes,

THE RIVERBANK

and most of the remaining pages are at least partially damaged. After carefully scrutinizing these pages, experts determine that it is likely there is not one manuscript here, but two, almost certainly written by different people. Your task, that I kindly allot to you in this thought experiment, is to divide the pages into two piles, one for each manuscript.

The idea behind the thought experiment is that the content of each page – what the writing on each page is about – will not be enough for you to distinguish between each manuscript, for much of this content is lost. What remains of this content may be substantially similar for both, so there is not enough of this remaining content to allow you to decisively adjudicate which page goes into which pile. To differentiate between manuscripts, you are going to have to rely on *style*. A difficult, but not impossible, undertaking. Suppose, for example, one of the manuscripts contains many sentences of this sort: 'We others who have long lost the more subtle of the physical senses have not even the proper terms to express an animal's intercommunication with his surroundings, living or otherwise, and have only the word "smell", for instance, to include the whole range of delicate thrills which murmur in the nose of the animal night and day, summoning, warning, inciting, repelling.' What can you tell from this? Most obviously, the sentence is long with subordinate clauses aplenty. By the time you get to the end of the sentence you might have forgotten what the beginning was about. A page with a sentence of this sort might, therefore, fall into one pile – the Kenneth Grahame pile.

THE BOOK OF MEMORY

Other pages, however, seem to be expressions of a rather different style. 'We others, deaf to the finer senses, can't even name the whispers that guide the beasts. "Smell" is all we've got, a blunt tool for a world of delicate dance. The animal knows, in its bones, the scent of danger, of love, of prey. We, blind and deaf, stumble through the dark. Home! That was the meaning of the familiar stench, of the stinking blankets that lay on the floor. The hands still tugged him, in this dream from which he had awakened. He must go south. There would be no surviving another winter here.' Probably not Kenneth Grahame, you can conclude. In fact, this was my best – but, I accept, still laughably poor – attempt to impersonate the style of Cormac McCarthy as a way of illustrating a certain point: namely, that it is possible to differentiate manuscripts based on style even in the absence of significant content. Even if you don't recognize the style as that of Cormac McCarthy you can still put this page in the non–Kenneth Grahame pile.

The eventual result of your labours, if you are sufficiently assiduous, would be two piles: two manuscripts which, although drastically incomplete, form recognizable wholes. They do so in the sense that the decision to allot a given page to one pile rather than the other is not an arbitrary or unprincipled one. Rather, it is a decision based on your analysis of the style of the pages in each pile, coupled with whatever content remains. The less content that remains – that is, the more pages that have been lost or damaged – the more your judgement must be based on style. You can make

THE RIVERBANK

mistakes, but on the other hand, you can also be right. And the fact that you can be right or wrong about this means that each pile has a genuine *identity* – an identity that we discern through its style.

If you can differentiate one manuscript from another, it is because you have, unconsciously at least, picked up on the various elements that go into a style of writing – the elements of literary style. These include, to name just a few: *vocabulary* (simple or complicated), *sentence structure* (long or short, subordinate clauses, fragmented or full), *figures of speech* (metaphors, similes, symbols, metonymy, personification), *perspective* (first, second, third, omniscient, limited omniscient, multiple inanimate, free indirect), *tone* (wistful, sarcastic, sardonic, ironic, detached, disappointed), *word colour* (alliteration, assonance, consonance, dissonance, rhythm), *dialogue* (yes or no, frequency), *paragraph structure* (short or long), *chapter structure* (short or long, organization), *characters* (function, method of introduction, development), *pace* (fast or slow, descriptive or action-orientated), *chronology* (organization of events, structural rhythm), *allusion* (employment of myths, symbols, other texts, historical personages and events), *experimentation* (stream-of-consciousness narratives, mixing of styles or genres, breaking of rules of grammar, unusual page layouts, onomatopoeia, unstable narrative perspectives), *metafictional techniques* (author as narrator, etc.).

These just scratch the surface of the elements of literary style – the things that go together, in varying combinations, to forge the style of a book. You don't notice these when you read – unless you pay them special attention because you are writing an academic paper or something like that – but on some level, you are aware of them. You are aware of them because this is what allows you to recognize a style and distinguish it from other styles. If you can distinguish pages written in the style of Kenneth Grahame from pages written in the style of Cormac McCarthy, this is because of your – implicit, unconscious – understanding of how stylistic elements combine together to yield a style.

12

RILKEAN STYLE

In the construction of a person, Rilkean memories play a role akin to that of literary style in the construction of a book. The identity of a book depends on both its content (what it is about, the story it tells) and its style (the way it expresses what it is about, the way it tells its story). The less content that remains, the more the identity of a book will be carried by its style. The same is true of a person. Our Rilkean memories bind us together, maintain each of us as a unified, unitary person when the content of our standard, episodic memories is lost. The less that remains of the content of their memories, the more a person becomes a style – an existential rather than a literary style.

The ability of Rilkean memories to play this person-maintaining role depends on how deeply they are entrenched and for how long they endure. In his memoir *The Story of a Life*, Aharon Appelfeld relates the seven years of his life he spent hiding from the Nazis in the woods of

THE BOOK OF MEMORY

Ukraine. From his account, here is a very good example of a Rilkean memory that is deeply entrenched and enduring: 'For years after the war, I did not walk in the middle of the pavement or path, but always close to the wall, always in the shade, always in a hurry like someone fleeing.' Here we seem to find both embodied and affective Rilkean memories. The memory is embodied in that it shows itself as a type of behaviour – walking in the shade, in a hurry. The memory is affective to the extent that it involves certain emotions or moods – a fundamental uneasiness, a horror of visibility – that underwrite his behaviour. These embodied and affective Rilkean memories are entrenched to the extent that they occur reliably – more or less whenever Appelfeld is given a choice of where to walk on a path. They are enduring to the extent that they persisted for many years after the war. The more entrenched and enduring a Rilkean memory is, the stronger its role will be in making someone the person they are.

My father was born around the same time as Appelfeld, although his childhood was a far happier one. However, Rilkean memories are indifferent to the nature of the remembered episodes. They spring as often from happy lives as they do from sad ones. In this respect, they are different from Freudian memories, which result from the repression of specifically unpleasant memories (although, as I mentioned earlier, Freud talked of repression of desires rather than of repression of memories), the result of the operations of a psychic defence mechanism. While some Rilkean

RILKEAN STYLE

memories may be Freudian, many Rilkean memories are not. Rilkean memories are far more widespread than their Freudian counterparts, and there is nothing necessarily defensive about them. In other words, even if there is such a thing as Freudian repressed memory, the category of Rilkean memory is much broader than that of Freudian memory.

Here is an example of what I am reasonably sure is a deeply entrenched and enduring Rilkean memory of my father. Grandpa Peter, as my sons briefly knew him, was born in December 1929, a couple of months after the stock market crash that heralded the Great Depression. He was always very frugal with money, but only in certain respects. When he retired, he was on one of those two-thirds-of-final-salary pensions that people of my generation can only dream about. He and my mother could live fairly comfortably. He enjoyed himself. He bought a boat, for example. And on one occasion, he decided without blinking to replace all the (rotting) windows in their house. But under certain eliciting conditions his reaction to even the smallest amount of fiscal outlay was very different. At that time, to cross the Cleddau Bridge – my parents retired to Pembrokeshire – required such an outlay: the princely sum of seventy-five pence. Whenever anyone suggested a trip across the bridge, his face took on the haunted look of a convict recently escaped from jail, who hears the first howls of the hounds in the distance.

If this emotion was a Rilkean memory, it would have been the result of intentional degradation of episodic memories from his early childhood during the Depression. Perhaps there was something about small financial outlays that triggered this reaction, since large financial outlays wouldn't have even been on the agenda in the early days of my father's life. Small financial outlays would have been a matter to be decided – and, presumably, disputed – daily. If this was a Rilkean memory, then it was *entrenched* and *enduring*, a reliable feature of my father's personality and spanning much of the second half of his life. This Rilkean memory had become part of my father's existential style.

Rilkean memories, especially those that are entrenched and enduring, encompass much of what people have in mind when they talk about a person's *character*. My favourite pre-Socratic philosopher, Heraclitus of Ephesus, once remarked: *character is destiny*. Character connects you to your future. Maybe it is and maybe it does. But more than that, and before that, *character is memory*, Rilkean memory. Rilkean memory is character in the deep historical sense, in that it pertains not to what you are now, but to how you came to be what you are now. Character can link you to a future by determining your destiny. But the character that is made of Rilkean memories connects you to your past – a past you thought you had forgotten but, in reality, could not forget.

The idea of literary style yields at least a partial answer to the question of what might bind together a literary work butchered by redactions. We are all, in our own way, suffering from catastrophic memory loss. The further back you travel into the book of memory, the larger the dark sea of redactions grows. However, this book of you has a style,

RILKEAN STYLE

no less than any other book – one that can help hold you together, as a unitary, unified whole, in the face of massive loss of content. 'Give style to your character,' Nietzsche once said. In a way, he was right, although his framing it as an injunction was misguided. Every one of us will give style to our character, whether we want to or not. We maintain ourselves in existence through a style bequeathed to us by our Rilkean memories.

Part Three

BRIGHT ISLANDS IN THE NIGHT

The sunless, redactional waters of Lethe are by no means undifferentiated. Look closer. You will see activity, unceasing and boundless. These currents, these whirlpools and gyres, waves and tidal races, are the Rilkean memories of Lethe. The Mediterranean has a style, and the Caribbean, the Southern Ocean and the Pacific. So too does this dark ocean of forgetting. We are more Lethe than we are the shining islands that remain. And in the dark currents of forgetting, one can discern the style of a man or a woman.

While the oil-black ocean may be the most obvious feature of the book of you, it is by no means its strangest. The strangest thing about this book is not its sunless tides but the islands that endure. The sands of these islands are shifting. They will betray you. Beware: these islands are not what they seem.

13

STENDHAL'S SYNDROME

'My heart was leaping wildly within me. What utterly childlike excitement!' Here, Stendhal, aka Marie-Henri Beyle, is (supposedly) describing his state of mind as the coach on which he is travelling descends from the Apennines into Florence, on his first visit to the city. On his arrival, he tells us, he rushed straight to the Basilica of Santa Croce, where, he relates, the 'tide of emotion' that overwhelmed him 'flowed so deep that it was scarce to be distinguished from religious awe'. The ultimate consequence of all of this was what has now become known as *Stendhal's syndrome*: dizziness, fainting, even hallucinations, when exposed to art – especially large quantities of art. As he emerged from the porch of Santa Croce, he claimed, he was 'seized with fierce palpitation of the heart'; the 'wellspring of life' dried up within him, and he walked 'in constant fear of falling to the ground'.

Ironically, if there is such a thing as Stendhal's syndrome,

THE BOOK OF MEMORY

Stendhal himself almost certainly did not suffer from it. These descriptions are taken from his book *Rome, Naples and Florence* – a book that was published in 1817 (with an expanded version published in 1826), but which describes events that took place in 1811, when Stendhal was plain old Marie-Henri Beyle, an aspiring writer from Grenoble who, with a view to broadening his mind through travel, had managed to attach himself to Napoleon's wandering army. Beyle, however, also bequeathed to us a journal written at the time of his travels in 1811, and this journal tells a very different story. Far from experiencing 'childlike excitement' as he descended into Florence, his journal tells us that he was 'overcome with fatigue, wet and jolted'. Instead of rushing straight to Santa Croce, as he tells us he did in 1817, he actually went to bed for the rest of the day at an inn, the Auberge d'Angleterre. The only reason he stayed in Florence was that the following day's coach to Rome was full. And the one the day after, and the one the day after that. Of his visit to Santa Croce, he does not even mention what you might expect him to mention – namely, Giotto's frescoes – although he does briefly mention the Niccolini Chapel that houses them. Nor, for that matter, does he mention any of the other of today's agreed-upon masterpieces. Of course, tastes change, but even so, not to have mentioned *any* of them?

One might be uncharitable and regard Beyle's journal entries as dissembling. Personally, being of a somewhat cynical bent, I think it more likely that he had a 'fertile imagination'. However, if you wanted to make a case for Beyle's integrity,

STENDHAL'S SYNDROME

it would be bolstered by an extensive body of scientific studies that has highlighted the extraordinary fragility and unreliability of memory. These studies indicate that the sort of discrepancies we find between Beyle's accounts of 1811 and 1817, even if these accounts were sincerely offered, are precisely what we should expect.

14

CHALLENGER

While it is difficult to overlook the fragility of memory in general – we have all forgotten far more than we remember – people used to think there was a certain type of memory that was unusually permanent and reliable. This was known as a *flashbulb memory*. The idea was that there was a special mechanism in the brain that, when triggered by an event that reaches a certain level of surprise and significance – the assassination of Kennedy, 9/11 etc. – would create a stable, permanent record of the details and circumstances of the event. Accordingly, flashbulb memories were regarded as especially reliable forms of memory.

This idea of the permanence and reliability of flashbulb memories was decisively debunked by Ulric Neisser and Nicole Harsch's now classic study of the 1986 *Challenger* explosion. *Challenger* was a space shuttle that exploded on 28 January 1986, a mere seventy-three seconds into its flight. The launch was watched by an atypically large number of

CHALLENGER

people – some 17 per cent of the US population – because of the presence on board of Christa McAuliffe, a high-school teacher who was the first participant in the Reagan administration's Teacher in Space Project.

The morning after the disaster, Neisser, a psychology professor at Emory University in Georgia, and Harsch, at that time his graduate assistant, distributed a short questionnaire to his class asking his students to describe how they had learned of the explosion, including where they were, what they were doing, who told them and who else was present. The completed questionnaires were put away until the freshmen of 1986 had become seniors in 1989. Neisser and Harsch then contacted those of the original participants who were still on campus. They filled out a questionnaire identical to the original and were also asked to rate their confidence in each of their memories. The results were striking. Here is one example. In 1986, RT gave this account of hearing the news:

> I was in my Religion class and some people walked in and started talking about [it]. I didn't know any details except that it had exploded and the schoolteacher's students had all been watching which I thought was so sad. Then after class I went to my room and watched the TV program talking about it and I got all the details from that.

RT's 1989 report, however, is rather different:

THE BOOK OF MEMORY

> When I first heard about the explosion I was sitting in my freshman dorm room with my roommate and we were watching TV. It came on a news flash and we were both totally shocked. I was really upset and I went upstairs to talk to a friend of mine and then I called my parents.

The first report was given less than twenty-four hours after the event, and therefore it is assumed to be relatively accurate. The second report diverges significantly. RT, however, recorded high confidence in her memories. She was far from alone in this – both in the inaccuracy of her flashbulb memories and in her confidence in their accuracy. GA, in 1986, reported that she was in the cafeteria when she heard the news, and it made her so sick she was unable to finish her lunch. In 1989, however, she reported, 'I was in my dorm room when some girl came running down the hall screaming, "The space shuttle just blew up."' On a scale of zero to seven – where zero meant that nothing was remembered correctly and seven meant that every aspect of the report was correct – eleven of the forty-four subjects scored zero, and five of those zeros nevertheless expressed high confidence in the accuracy of their memories.

In the spring of 1990, Neisser and Harsch conducted a follow-up. When shown their 1986 responses, none of the students was inclined to change their 1989 account. Many of the low-accuracy, high-confidence responders were shocked, but did not back down. A few even argued that they must have been wrong the first time (on the day after the event) because they were surely right now. These results have been replicated in a number of other studies. In general, the feature that most reliably accompanies flashbulb memories is a high degree of confidence shown by people in them, rather than accuracy.

Neisser and Harsch's study is targeted on what I earlier called the *episodicity* of the memories, rather than their semantic aspect. After all, no one forgot that the *Challenger* exploded. This semantic memory seems immune to the kinds of revision identified in their study. Rather, what are susceptible to revision are the features of these memories that make them episodic: what one was doing when one heard the news, with whom one was doing it, where one was, how one first heard the news and so on. Your flashbulb memories are ones whose episodicity you are really confident about – that is, you are confident about the features that make the memory episodic. But this confidence turns out to be misplaced. There is a significant chance that you are mistaken about these episodic details. Despite your confidence in them, these island sentences in the books of you – even the especially luminescent flashbulb islands – are likely to be inaccurate in a variety of ways, ranging from the misplacement or misalignment of a few details at one end of the spectrum to much more dramatic falsity at the other. These results have been replicated so many times it is difficult to doubt them. The important question is not whether our memories – yours, mine and everyone else's – are surprisingly inaccurate, but why they should be this way.

15

MAKING AND REMAKING MEMORIES

Endemic unreliability is not an accidental feature of memory but a consequence of its underlying neurobiology – the brain processes that go on when we retrieve our memories. The crux of the issue is that the way in which memories are first created and the way in which they are later retrieved are more similar than has, until recently, been realized. The creation of a memory is known as *encoding*. For a memory to be encoded, a set of connections must be established between neurons. These connections will underwrite a set of *activity dependencies*. An activity dependency is a relation between neurons in which the firing of one neuron has certain implications for the firing of other neurons to which that neuron is connected. If the connection is excitatory, the firing of one neuron will cause the firing of the other neurons to which it is connected. (Suppose, for example, activity in one neuron represents smoke. The firing of this neuron may cause the firing of another neuron, activity in which is supposed to represent fire. If so, the connection between the two neurons is said to be excitatory.) If the connection is inhibitory, on the other hand, the firing of one neuron will inhibit or dampen the firing of connected neurons. (Activation of a neuron whose job is to represent water may reduce – figuratively, dampen – the likelihood of activity in the neuron dedicated to representing fire.) These relationships of excitement and inhibition can be further nuanced through the introduction of thresholds, where the excitation or inhibition of neuronal activity kicks in only after a certain threshold of activity has been reached in the original, stimulating neuron. (For example, the smoke neuron must be firing at a certain frequency or amplitude before the fire neuron becomes activated.) This establishing of networks of connected neurons – circuits in the brain – is known as *long-term potentiation*.

Long-term potentiation is, essentially, a construction process. At the core of any neuron is a long, cylindrical tube known as an *axon*. At one end of the neuron, the axon culminates in what is known as the *axon terminal*. At the other end is the *dendrite*, a collection of small, twig-like projections. The function of this dendritic end of the neuron is to receive input. The function of the axon terminal is to supply output. Communication between neurons occurs when the dendritic end of one neuron becomes linked to the axonal terminal of another neuron. The point of connection between the two is known as the *synapse*. At the synapse, the axon terminal and the dendritic end of the two neurons come into close proximity, and electrical and chemical messages can be sent across the small gap between them.

A memory is first formed as a short-term memory. Its future prospects require it to be converted into a more stable long-term counterpart. For this to happen, new connections between neurons need to be created. This is done by way of a series of gene activations and the resulting protein synthesis. The protein synthesis can have several distinct results. New receptor cells might be built at the dendritic end of the neuron. Alternatively, the amount of chemical neurotransmitters used to send messages across the synapse may be increased. New ion channels – proteins that create an opening in a cell membrane that allows ions (positively or negatively charged particles) to pass through – may be created, and this also increases connectivity between neurons. The result of this protein synthesis is that hitherto unconnected neurons now become connected. The result is the *consolidation* of a memory into long-term form.

Consolidation is the process whereby long-term memories are first created. When an episode is first experienced, it enters short-term memory. Short-term memories are relatively ephemeral and labile – that is, vulnerable to interference from extraneous factors. The function of consolidation is to convert memories of this sort into something more robust and stable. These more robust descendants are long-term memories.

MAKING AND REMAKING MEMORIES

Consolidation is the process by which a long-term memory is first created or encoded. Until very recently, it was thought that the process whereby a previously created long-term memory is *retrieved* is very different. The most significant discovery in memory research in the last half a century is that the encoding and the retrieval of memories are much more similar than was previously thought. In particular, when a memory is retrieved, it returns, in effect, to the unstable labile state characteristic of short-term memory. It must then undergo a process of *reconsolidation*. The endemic inaccuracy of memory is a consequence of this.

Proteins are the basis of any new biological construction, including the building of neural connections in the ways described above. Thus, consolidation of a short-term memory can occur only if new proteins are created: that is, if protein synthesis occurs. It has recently become clear that the same process of protein synthesis occurs both when long-term memories are encoded *and* when they are retrieved. Karim Nader and colleagues tested the hypothesis that protein synthesis was involved in retrieving memories by blocking protein synthesis during memory retrieval in rats. Several rats were conditioned to associate a loud noise with a painful electric shock. On hearing the noise, the rats exhibited fear behaviour (freezing in place, etc.). After several weeks of conditioning, Nader injected the rats with a protein-synthesis inhibitor – anisomycin. When the loud noise was played again, the memory had seemingly disappeared. The rats no longer displayed fear behaviour when the noise was played, and this absence of fear behaviour continued after the effects of the protein inhibitor had worn off.

The conclusion Nader drew is that if the requisite proteins cannot be created during the act of retrieval, then the original memory will cease to exist. This conclusion was supported by the identification – by Todd Sacktor and colleagues – of the crucial protein involved in both the formation and the retrieval of memories. This is PKMzeta – a form of kinase C protein. PKMzeta is prevalent in the synaptic connections that link neurons together, and without it these connections will become unstable and eventually disappear. But PKMzeta also plays a crucial role in the retrieval of memories. If a PKMzeta inhibitor is injected into rats prior to the retrieval of a memory, the memory will disappear just as the memories did in Nader's rats.

The biological and chemical processes that occur when a memory is encoded and when it is later retrieved are substantially similar. After encoding, memories are consolidated. After retrieval, memories must be *reconsolidated*. The importance of the fact that remembering requires reconsolidation cannot be overstated. It is, ultimately, this that underlies the divergence between the 1986 and 1989 responses of the subjects in Neisser and Harsch's *Challenger* study. The implications, however, run deeper than this and ultimately call into question the way in which our memories connect us to our past.

16

THE BEACHES OF MEMORY

The first casualty of the discovery of memory reconsolidation – there will be more – is the *storage* or *imprinting* model of memory. In the *Theaetetus*, Plato compared memory to a block of wax:

> I would have you imagine, then, that there exists in the mind of man a block of wax ... Let us say that this tablet is a gift of Memory, the mother of the Muses; and that when we wish to remember anything which we have seen, or heard, or thought in our own minds, we hold the wax to the perceptions and thoughts, and in that material receive the impression of them as from the seal of a ring; and that we remember and know what is imprinted as long as the image lasts; but when the image is effaced, or cannot be taken, then we forget and do not know.

Before the discovery of reconsolidation, accepted accounts

of memory were heavily indebted to this Platonic picture whereby short-term memories are formed while the wax is still soft, and as such are labile – vulnerable to outside influences that might distort (smudge) them. Quickly, however, the wax hardens – consolidates – yielding robust, stable and relatively permanent long-term memories.

If this model were correct, distortions of memory would be largely confined to soft, labile short-term memories. Once these have hardened into long-term memories, they would be far more resistant to revision. This, however, is incompatible with the sorts of memory distortion described by Neisser and Harsch. After all, by the time the students were first asked to describe their experiences of the *Challenger* disaster (the following day), long-term memories had already formed. The discrepancy between their earlier and later testimonies is, therefore, indicative of a discrepancy between two long-term memories.

The neurobiological evidence, however, steers us in a very different direction. Put in terms of Plato's model, we might think of memory retrieval as always involving a re-softening of the wax. When a memory is recalled, it once again enters the unstable, labile state characteristic of short-term memory and is now susceptible to distortion. That is no guarantee that the memory will be distorted. The wax might re-harden in the same form. But the possibility of distortion is always there in every act of retrieval.

Augustine had a similar model of memory to Plato which only differed in superficial details. Instead of wax,

THE BEACHES OF MEMORY

Augustine preferred the storehouse metaphor:

> I come to the fields and vast palaces of memory, where are the treasures of all kinds of objects brought to it by sense perception ... When I am in this storehouse, I ask that it produce what I want to recall, and immediately certain things come out, some require a longer search and have to be drawn out from as it were more recondite receptacles ... Memories of earlier events give way to those which followed, and as they pass are stored away available for retrieval when I want them.

Like Plato's wax model, we now know that this picture is inaccurate. It would, perhaps, be more accurate if pulling an item from one of the receptacles of the storehouse involved squeezing it out of a narrow aperture, and so required the item to first become soft and malleable – and potentially distorted by the act of retrieval.

Plato had his wax, and Augustine had his storehouse. I, on the other hand – informed by a knowledge of reconsolidation that Plato and Augustine could not have had – have my shining islands in the Ocean of Lethe. Every time you walk on the sands of these islands, there is a possibility you will change them. Typically, when you walk on the golden beaches of memory you change them. At first, you might leave nothing more than gentle, barely discernible footprints in the sand. But with each visit these footsteps grow deeper. The contours of the beach slowly change. The

THE BOOK OF MEMORY

sand slowly erodes. Patterns of vegetation are changed. The island mutates. Restoration is required to return the island to its original, unspoiled state. But how do you remember what the island used to be like? Your memory of the island is the island itself, in this new and altered state. You cannot get outside your memories of the past to the past itself.

17

INVITATIONS

The phenomenon of reconsolidation means that every time it is retrieved, the possibility of revision – minor, major or somewhere in between – haunts every episodic memory. Indeed, the possibility lies at the heart of what makes a memory episodic. You might think of any episodic memory as an invitation. Every episodic memory invites you to complete it.

As I have already mentioned, in Neisser and Harsch's *Challenger* study there is one feat of recall that seems immune to revision: no one forgot that *Challenger* exploded. This is a semantic memory, a memory of a fact. The possibility of revision that haunts episodic memory pertains to what I earlier called the *episodicity* of the memory. The episodicity of a memory consists in the features that make it episodic. In the imagined Vesuvian time-travel scenario discussed earlier, the episodicity of this memory was the sight of the massive ash cloud, the stench of sulphur in the air, the ear-splitting sound of the explosion. If, courtesy of my time-travel machine, I had these experiences, then my memory of the eruption of Vesuvius would be an episodic one rather than the merely semantic memory that it in fact is. The experiences of sight, sounds and smells would make the memory an episodic one. Together, they would make up the episodicity of this memory.

The same is true in the *Challenger* case. I don't have an episodic memory of the *Challenger* explosion. My memory of this event is, it seems, purely semantic. What would make it episodic is an array of experiential details – where I was when I heard of the explosion or saw it on TV, what I was doing at the time, who I was with, how the event made me feel, and so on. These are, of course, the kinds of experiences targeted in Neisser and Harsch's questionnaire. To the extent that it is these features that vary across time – and, to reiterate, no one who participated in the study forgot that *Challenger* exploded – it is the episodicity of an episodic memory that becomes vulnerable upon recall. The features that make a memory episodic – experiences of 'sitting in my dorm room', of being 'in my Religion class', or of a 'girl ... running down the hall screaming' – are the ones liable to change upon retrieval of that memory.

These kinds of experiential details make a memory episodic in a simple, but striking, way: they place the person who has these experiences *in* the memory itself. Suppose, contrary to fact, I did episodically remember the *Challenger* explosion. I was, let us suppose, in the Graduate Common

INVITATIONS

Room at Jesus College, Oxford mid-morning when I saw the event on TV. There were people around me, and I remember talking to them about what was happening. I remember thinking how sad it was. (In this imagined memory, there is no one running up and down the hall screaming, perhaps because this was Oxford in the 1980s and, I seem to remember, we didn't do that sort of thing.) These experiential details transform the episode from a simple event that happened in a given place and at a given time into an episode that was formerly witnessed by me. That is what the addition of these episodic details does. It presents – portrays – the episode precisely as one that I formerly experienced. These experiential details, if I had them, would make my memory episodic, not because of what they are in themselves but because of what they do. Because of these details, the *Challenger* explosion is presented to me precisely *as* an episode *I* have formerly experienced. These experiences, in this sense, insert me into the memory.

The presence of the *I*, of the remembering self, is a non-negotiable part of episodic memory. This is an event that *I* formerly witnessed. This is an event that happened to *me*. This is an event that *I* once orchestrated. The presence of the self in memory is, as I mentioned earlier, known as autonoesis. For autonoesis to occur, certain experiential details must be provided, where these details have the function of presenting an episode *as* one I have formerly experienced. The provision of these sorts of details, details that have precisely this purpose, we might call the *completion* of the memory. Every episodic memory both invites and, indeed, requires completion – every such memory is an invitation to completion in this sense, and without this completion the memory cannot be episodic. If a memory is not completed, it can be nothing more than a semantic memory.

However, as we now know, the experiential details required to complete an episodic memory are shifting and labile – vulnerable to interference during the act of recall. It is precisely these experiential details that must be rebuilt – completed – in the act of recall. Therefore, while this completion may be accurate, often it is not. As the Neisser/Harsch study shows, this completion may be far less accurate than we naively assume. GA reports, 'I was in my dorm room when some girl came running down the hall screaming, "The space shuttle just blew up."' She has supplied experiential details required to make the memory an episodic one. But these details, we are in a strong position to suppose, do not reflect the details of the experiences she actually had in 1986. Her memory is still episodic. There was an episode. She experienced it. And she remembers it now as an episode she formerly experienced. She has an episodic memory, but an inaccurate one.

You don't have to remember an event episodically – just ask R.B. But if you do, you had better be willing to fill in the kind of experiential details required for an episode to be experienced as one you have formerly encountered. You might think of remembering as analogous to the movie industry. 'Here is a suggestion, a theme, an overarching plot – spacecraft

INVITATIONS

explodes – now you fill in the details.' A studio executive overseeing several hard-working, underpaid screenwriters: that is the essence of episodic remembering. You don't have to work here, but if you want to you had better be prepared to fill in the plot details. It is a strange sort of invitation, perhaps, straddling elements of an invitation and an offer that can't be refused, but I gather the movie industry is a little like that. Episodic memories both invite and, if they are to be episodic memories, demand completion, and this completion is, to say the least, not an entirely reliable process.

What should we make of the endemic unreliability of episodic memory? This unreliability is the result of the fact that when memories are retrieved they must be reconsolidated. Why did the brain hit upon this way of doing it? Is it an accident? A design flaw in the brain's strategy for remembering? Many think so, but I suspect not. In fact, I suspect that reconsolidation, together with the resulting instability of episodic memory, is a crucial part of remembering episodically in the sense that there are some memories we can only have if we change them – amend or transform the features that make them episodic. In other words, sometimes the details I need to supply for the memory to qualify as episodic must be inaccurate ones – because it is only in inaccurate form that I can have this memory. I haven't argued for this yet. I shall do so in the coming pages. I shall try to convince you there are some memories that can qualify as episodic only if they are inaccurate. Inaccuracy is, in these cases, a precondition – a sine qua non – of remembering.

THE BOOK OF MEMORY

My suspicion, then, is that *all* memories are susceptible to revision because *some* memories will have to be revised – precisely so we can have them. The problem is that we do not know in advance which memories are going to require revision. Indeed, which memories these are will almost certainly change with time and circumstance. Therefore, the possibility of revision – the susceptibility to alteration – will haunt every memory. For a good example of a memory that has been revised in this way – and that had to be revised in this way – we might mentally travel back in time to the early hours of the morning of 26 May 1965.

18

THE FACE OF MY FATHER

It is so difficult to trap memory in a lie. To do so, it seems, you would need to be able to compare memory with the past. But your memory is your only record of the past, and you can never stand outside memory to see the past as it really was. It is difficult, therefore, to trap memory in this way, but not impossible. For there are some memories that we have that we know must be inaccurate. I have a memory of my father's face that is of just this sort.

My father died more than a decade ago. My children were still young when he died and their memories of him seem largely restricted to his being a convenient foil for making fun of me. 'You look like Grandpa Peter, Dad!' That's after every haircut I ever had. Before long there was further innovation: 'Baldilocks!' or 'Balderella!' Not that there is anything at all wrong with it, but, for the record, I am not bald, and probably will not become bald. Neither was Grandpa Peter, for that matter. As far as I know, there is no

THE BOOK OF MEMORY

male-pattern baldness in the family. My hair, like my father's hair before me, is merely undergoing some unavoidable thinning due to age-related testosterone depletion. Amid the jibes, I can take a smidgen of grim solace in the knowledge that my sons have that to look forward to as well.

I miss my father, and perhaps because of this I have found my memory turning towards him quite a bit in the years since his death. There is one memory in particular that has intrigued me in a variety of ways – an episode that lies at the very limits of my memory. (So near the limits, in fact, that I doubt it is a memory, at least not *my* memory. But that is a topic for later.) The memory is of the face of my father. In particular, it is a memory of certain transformations undergone by my father's face in the early hours of the morning (BST) of 26 May 1965. I know the date retrospectively, of course: this was the date of the second Muhammad Ali–Sonny Liston fight, that took place in Lewiston, Maine. The order of events, apparently, transpired thus: shortly before the fight commenced, the two-year-old me woke up, restless and hungry. My father, perhaps realizing that the only way to placate me was via some warm milk, hurried off to heat some up in a saucepan on the kitchen stove. There were no microwaves back then, of course. When he returned, the fight was already over. Ali had knocked Liston out inside one hundred seconds, with a punch so fast that many had trouble seeing it. But that is not important. What is important is my father's face: a study in confusion, flitting between the TV screen and me – as if I were somehow responsible

THE FACE OF MY FATHER

for the events unfolding, in black and white, before his disbelieving eyes. What is going on? Are they showing the conclusion of their first fight, in Miami? Confusion slowly turns to suspicion: a hypothesis – had I fiddled with the TV in some way? Suspicion transforms to grim resignation: he had missed it! And resignation turns to happiness: my father was a great admirer of Ali's intelligence and skill.

I chose this episode for two reasons. First, I have very good reasons for supposing that an episode of this sort did occur. Let's face it, my dad wasn't going to let *that* go: the time I robbed him of the opportunity – except in numerous replays, of course – to witness Ali knocking out Liston! I was never allowed to hear the end of it. So, we are not dealing with confabulation here – it is not a case of apparently remembering something that never really happened. Second, there are very good reasons for thinking I could not have originally experienced this episode in the way I now remember it. This is so in two ways, actually, both of them important. Here, I am going to talk about just one of them: the apparent *age* of my father's face.

When this fight took place, my father would have been a relatively young man – thirty-five years of age, I believe. However, the face I remember, slowly transforming from confusion to suspicion to grim resignation to joy, is the face of an old man. It is the face he wore in his final years. Why would this be? To understand why I would remember my father's face as old, it is necessary to understand the paucity of photographs at that time – a paucity that will be difficult to grasp for those who have grown up in the selfie age: an age of vast continents of photographs, untethered to the physical earth, drifting, largely unwatched, through cyberspace. Things weren't always like this. Mobile phones, obviously, hadn't been invented in 1965. Neither had cyberspace. There was a device called a Polaroid – a camera that would print out a photograph roughly, if my memory serves me well, a minute or two after you had taken it. You had to be careful how you held it when it came out: like short-term memory, it was still wet and easily smudged. But even Polaroids hadn't made it to South Wales in 1965. Therefore, making a photograph was a protracted, wearisome affair involving a camera that wouldn't work a significant proportion of the time, a high risk of exposure when you removed the film from the camera, a trip to a pharmacist (the 'chemist', as we called them back then), and a wait of approximately two weeks while the photos were developed. Attrition rates were high: you'd be lucky to end up with half of the photos you'd actually taken. As a result of these obstacles, people couldn't be bothered – not often, anyway. Photographs were something reserved for special occasions: Christmas, birthdays, holidays – that kind of thing. My mum and dad were not averse to capturing their children in celluloid, but they certainly weren't going to go through the required rigmarole to take photographs of themselves. As a result, photographs of my father were few and far between. In fact, I don't think I saw any photographs of him as a young man until after he died.

With this historical context in mind, consider what would

THE FACE OF MY FATHER

have happened if, in my memory, the face slowly transforming from suspicion to joy were the face of my father as a young man. In such circumstances, there would be a significant chance I wouldn't recognize him. 'Who is this strange man that I remember?' would certainly be a possible – and perhaps not unlikely – reaction. Memory is not like this.

Don't get me wrong. There are certain circumstances in which I might have a memory of this latter sort. Suppose, contrary to fact, my father had abandoned us shortly after the events of this night unfolded, and I never saw him again. In these counterfactual circumstances, I might very well have had a memory of this sort, of a face I did not know but which seemed vaguely familiar, undergoing certain sorts of emotional transformations. But the memory I describe now is not this. What I remember is precisely my father's face – and I remember it *as* my father's face rather than the face of an unfamiliar man who just happens to be my father. I remember the face *as* my father's face transforming from confusion to suspicion to resignation to happiness. But I had not seen this face of 1965 for many, many years, and so would not have recognized it, at least not with the immediacy required of this memory of the face of my father. (A little like R.B., I might, for example, have had to work out who this person was through a process of inference.) Therefore, I had to change the face of my father – to make his face old rather than young – in order to be able to remember this face as my father's face.

I could not, of course, in 1965 have experienced my father's face as the face of an old man. That is something

THE BOOK OF MEMORY

I later added to the memory. The memory is, accordingly, inaccurate. However, what is crucial is that the inaccuracy of the memory is a precondition of my having it. If I hadn't altered the memory in this way, then it would not have been a memory – or it would have been a different memory. The memory, such as it is, could only exist in inaccurate form. This is how it is with memories sometimes. If we just focus on reconsolidation – the neurobiological processes involved in retrieving a memory – then it is tempting to view revision of the past as an accidental, and regrettable, feature of the process of remembering – a flaw in the way we remember. *If only the brain had come up with a better strategy*, we might be tempted to think. But I don't think it is a flaw at all. Sometimes we have to revise our memories – as I altered, in my memory, the age of my father's face – precisely so we can remember them. Sometimes we absolutely have to change what we remember because if we did not, we couldn't remember it. The *possibility* of revision haunts every memory because the *necessity* of revision haunts some of them – and we don't, in advance, know which ones these will be. Whenever we remember, therefore, we must be ready, willing and able to change the memory to whatever degree is necessary for us to remember it.

We change our memories in order to stay in them. If something is to qualify as an episodic memory, then what is remembered must be presented as something I have previously experienced, orchestrated or otherwise encountered. Sometimes altering the episode is necessary to achieve this.

THE FACE OF MY FATHER

I had to change the face of my father in my memory because if I hadn't, I wouldn't have recognized it as the face of my father. And if I did not recognize this face as the face of my father, then I would not have remembered this episode – in which his face transformed in the way I have described – as an episode that *I* formerly witnessed. Without this it would not have been an episodic memory. We are, all of us, in our memories, and that is why we need to change them. We change them precisely to keep up with the changes in us. Memories therefore bear the indelible stamp of the person who has them. Our fingerprints are all over our memories.

My fingerprints, in this sense, consist in the changes I have imposed on the episode to make it something I can remember. I call these changes my 'fingerprints' because they are reliable indicators of me, my circumstances and, fundamentally, my *history*. If, for example, more photographs of my father as a young man had existed, I probably would not have had to alter the episode in this way. If my youthful powers of visual imagery and my ability to fix these images into visual memories had been more acute – if, in other words, I had benefited from the highly superior autobiographical memory (HSAM) I mentioned earlier, eliminating the need for photographs – then, again, I might not have needed to transform the episode. But given the specific circumstances of my history – given things were the way they were – I did have to change the episode in the way I have described.

Our thinking about catastrophic memory loss is overly

THE BOOK OF MEMORY

influenced by what we might think of as the *mosaic model*. Imagine a mosaic, comprising thousands, tens of thousands or hundreds of thousands of tiny tiles. Collectively, these tiles tell a story, but slowly the tiles become lost. The story becomes more and more difficult to comprehend. Eventually, too many tiles are lost, and the story irretrievably breaks down.

This, however, is not the right picture of memory loss. It would be a better picture if we acknowledged that each of the tiles that remains bears the indelible stamp of the person whose story it tells. It is a strange stamp, evident only to the subject of the story and invisible to all others, because only an invisible stamp will do.

Embossed on each of my memories is the stamp of Mark Rowlands, but the stamp is a subtle one. It is not one of those stamps that you'd dip in blue ink and press onto some document to indicate a form of proprietorship, or a stamp on your hand that gets you back into a nightclub. That sort of stamp would not work. It would no more show that the memory is mine than the corresponding stamp on a photograph would show that the photograph is mine. Someone might have mistakenly placed the stamp there or might be trying to trick me. Some stamps are far more subtle. They are as much about what is not there as they are about what is. The face of my father as a young man is no longer in this memory. This is my stamp. The stamp I have placed on this memory is to be found in the way I have transformed it from the original scene, transformed it precisely so I can remember it. The

THE FACE OF MY FATHER

memory bears the indelible – even though invisible – stamp of me. On all my memories there is the stamp of me. This stamp consists in the changes I have made to remembered episodes precisely so that I am able to remember them. Whether modest or immense, the stamp is always a subtle one. You cannot see it, but if you are lucky, and if you think hard enough, you can work out that it is there. For our episodic memories, only the most subtle of stamps will work.

We all place our stamp on our memories. Transforming memories in this way so that we might keep them, as I did with my memory of my father's face, is by no means uncommon. But the changes we have wrought are always veiled, for we cannot step outside these memories to see the past. Understanding that they have been changed – that we ourselves have changed them – is something that cannot be observed – it can only be inferred. If you want to find these memories in your own life, the most obvious place to begin your search is with *field* memories that have become *observer* memories. Perhaps you fell out of a tree when you were ten years old. At the time you would have experienced the rush of air and the forlorn embrace of the leaves and branches as you rushed by. This would be a field memory. You are the centre of this memory: the tree, the branches, the ground all revolve around you. You are the centre of the memory just as you were the centre of the original experience of falling. But it is quite likely that you now remember this episode very differently. It is common for field memories to transform, with age, into observer memories, in which you picture yourself falling from the tree as someone else – an observer – might have seen you. You remember the episode from the outside. You can easily infer that you could not have had these experiences as you fell – visual experiences of you falling as if seen from afar. Yet this is the way you now remember the event. It is not clear why this happens. But it does, and sometimes an observer memory is all that remains of what was once a field memory. With the memory of my father's face, we have something extra. We can understand not only that it has been changed, but also why it had to be changed. I could not have continued to have this memory without it being changed. I have not yet finished with this memory of my father's face. As yet, we have only scratched its surface.

Part Four

NEGOTIATING WITH THE PAST

The past is always a matter for the most delicate negotiation. To walk the bright sands of the islets of remembrance is to change them. But when dealing with the past, you can never stand outside your memories and compare what they are now with what they once were. You cannot remember how the islands used to be precisely because these islands – as they are now – are your memory.

You can reach the past only by negotiation. In negotiation, you work out how the past must have been if the present is to make any sense. You reconstruct the past and then remember your reconstruction.

Sometimes it is you who negotiates your own past. But it need not be you. This is the crowning realization, and in it lies a path. The path is a sunlit one that wends its way

THE BOOK OF MEMORY

upwards from the beach, through the pine woods, and onwards and forever upwards, through cow-parsleyed fields. At the end of this path you will find life everlasting. I hope you won't be disappointed.

19

EARTHQUAKE

If you were a book, you would be a book of memories. The idea that your memories make you who you are is a common one, in my profession at least. They are probably not the whole story of you, but it is difficult to deny that they are a significant part of that story. You are more than a specious 'now'. You are more than a now that 'goes by so quick you can hardly catch it going'. But the future is only a promise, a possibility, and as such is entirely diaphanous. With the past, there is the solidity of the having been. The past is solid and dense. The future is insubstantial, as light as a feather. The past is, therefore, more real, just as a solid, flesh-and-bone human is more real than an apparition. It is your past that makes you who you are. And your past is retained only in memories. If you were a book, therefore, you would be a book of memories. The problem is that memories are turning out to be much stranger than you might have thought. Far from being accurate representations of a past that formed you, they are more like unprincipled editorial intrusions designed to help you make sense of the present. The book of you is starting to look far less like an autobiography and far more like a self-help book. In its pages one finds not so much descriptions of the past, but rather negotiations with it.

Earlier, I compared episodic memory to the activities of a studio executive overseeing some hard-working screenwriters. The exec gives them an overarching theme. Studio execs being highly conservative creatures, this will probably be a combination of two successful precursors. The screenwriters fill in the details. The result will probably be horribly derivative but commercially attractive, starring someone like Dwayne Johnson in something like *San Andreas*. This analogy might, I think usefully, be pushed further. After all, it is not as if the screenwriters, once given their brief, have free rein. They are going to have to go back to the exec with their ideas. Perhaps he will like them. Perhaps he won't. Perhaps he will instruct them to think again. Particularly brave screenwriters might try to convince the exec of their vision for how the story should be filled in. Perhaps he will be swayed. Perhaps he will fire them and bring in someone else to do the job. The filling in of the details of the plot is often a matter of detailed *negotiation*. Memory completion – the filling in of experiential details necessary for an event to be recalled episodically – is one thing. All episodic memory requires this. But how the completion is to be achieved, and the form this completion takes, can often be the subject of delicate *negotiation*. Who is the negotiator, the one

EARTHQUAKE

conducting the negotiations, you might ask? It can be you. But it doesn't always have to be.

After the *Challenger* study, Neisser and colleagues conducted another study along the same lines. The focus of this second study was a sizeable earthquake that shook Northern California on 17 October 1989. The study was made up of three groups. First, there was a control group, comprising students at Emory University in Atlanta, a little over 2,000 miles away, who were interviewed soon after they had heard news of the earthquake. Second, there were students at the University of California, Berkeley, who had experienced the earthquake, but in a fairly mild form. These students were interviewed a couple of days after the event and were asked to describe their experiences: where they were when the earthquake hit, what they were doing at the time, and so on. A third group of students at the University of California, Santa Cruz – where the impact of the earthquake was much greater than it had been at Berkeley – were, due to difficult post-earthquake logistics, interviewed only after a couple of weeks had passed. All three groups were retested after eighteen months.

The Atlanta control group exhibited the sort of memory degradation evident in the *Challenger* study. By the time of the retest, serious errors had started to appear in these students' memories. Both California groups, in stark contrast, were near perfect in their recall after eighteen months. This might seem to support a traditional flashbulb model, according to which the strong emotional content of the experiences would burn the memories permanently and indelibly into their long-term-memory system. However, the evidence contradicts this conclusion. In the experiment, students were asked to rate their level of emotional arousal. Remember, the impact of the earthquake was much greater in Santa Cruz than in Berkeley, and therefore the emotional arousal of the students in Santa Cruz was greater than that of the Berkeley students. This was reflected in the reports of the students. Many of the Berkeley students barely registered the earthquake – minor earthquakes, for them, being largely 'old hat'. Reported levels of arousal were higher in the Santa Cruz students. According to the prediction of the traditional flashbulb model of memory, the Santa Cruz group should have had more accurate memories than their Berkeley counterparts. In fact, the accuracy of the reported memories was the same for the Berkeley and Santa Cruz groups. Contrary to the flashbulb model, there was no correlation between reported arousal and subsequent accuracy.

Why is it that the Berkeley students, many of whom barely noticed the earthquake, should have had such accurate memories? Neisser's answer: *talking*. If you are a person who has first-hand experience of a major earthquake – and few in other parts of the country are going to understand that what may be major in Santa Cruz may not be so major seventy-five miles away in Berkeley – then you are a person worth talking to. Relatives and friends will almost certainly call you to find out what you were doing when the earthquake struck, how you survived, what you were feeling and so on.

EARTHQUAKE

As a result, you find yourself telling this story over and over again. Your memories become *externalized* in the form of spoken reports. Written reports would probably work too. It is externalization that is the key, not the specific form it takes. (If emails had existed at the time, I suspect the writing and re-writing of the same story would have had a similar effect.) The effect of externalizing the memory in this way is pronounced even if you have nothing, really, to remember. Three subjects in the Berkeley area had not even noticed the earthquake while it was happening, but still – a year and a half later – knew exactly where they were and what they were doing while not noticing it.

On the face of it, Neisser's conclusion seems rather comforting. Memory, we now know, is endemically unreliable. But now we have discovered there are things we can do to mitigate the baleful effects of reconsolidation. Externalizing our memories – telling people about them – is a way of counteracting the inaccuracy of memory. It is a way of fixing memories that, in the act of recall, would otherwise become soft and pliable again. We might think of externalized verbal reports as providing an extra layer of security for our memories, buttressing them against the ravages of reconsolidation and the resulting inaccuracy. This is good news, surely? Robinson Crusoe might have had trouble with his memories, but those of us who have someone to talk to are in a much better boat.

The comfort provided by this idea, however, is only illusory. If you find it comforting, this is likely to be because

THE BOOK OF MEMORY

you have neglected to distinguish between two very different things: the *fixing* of a memory and the *accuracy* of a memory. By talking about our memories, we can fix them in stable form. But this will result in accurate memories only if what we say is true or accurate. Adding another layer of 'security' to our memories, in the form of a verbal report, changes nothing. In fact, it merely relocates our original problem. The original problem was placing an accuracy check on memories that, we have good reason to think, are likely to be unreliable. Externalized reports – essentially, self-testimony – merely push that problem back a step. Now we have the problem of placing an accuracy check on our testimony. There might be all sorts of reasons why what we tell ourselves and others about what happened diverges from what actually happened. If our spoken testimony has the immense power to lock in our memories in stable form, that power is truly worrying, because stability does not entail accuracy. We can be locking in memories that have been rendered inaccurate precisely because our testimony was inaccurate. We are supposed to police our memories by talking about them. But who is to police what it is that we say about our memories?

Nietzsche once wrote, '"I did that," says my memory. "I cannot have done that," says my pride. Eventually, memory yields.' Perhaps Nietzsche is right. Perhaps our memories are routinely sacrificed at the altar of self-aggrandizement. But perhaps this happens only rarely. How common a phenomenon this is is an empirical question, one that can be

EARTHQUAKE

answered only by detailed – empirical – studies. If Nietzsche is right, this would be an example of a negotiation with the past, although of a fairly crude, take-it-or-leave-it variety. 'You did this,' says memory. 'I'll see your offer,' says pride, 'and respond with a counter-offer: I didn't do it. That's my final offer by the way.' While crude, the general contours of this sort of negotiation with the past are clear enough. The past is a certain way. You don't like this way. And so you negotiate with the past until it assumes a more pleasing form. Negotiation with the past, however, does not have to be as nakedly self-serving as this. Sometimes we negotiate with the past not because we don't like it and want to change it, but because we don't understand it and want to make sense of it.

20

SUPER PIECE OF CRICKET, THAT!

The kind of negotiation with the past I am interested in is of the latter variety – namely, an attempt to understand what happened in the past rather than to substitute a desired version of the past. Here is an example. Early in the September of 1978, in the ancient city of Bath, my cricketing career reached its zenith – an apogee with respect to which the rest of my career was, I'm sad to say, an anaemic disappointment. The fifteen-year-old me was facing an adult and – to my inexperienced eyes at least – frighteningly fast bowler from the Lansdowne Cricket Club. Here is how I remember my short-lived ascension to greatness. The ball sent in my direction was drifting down the leg side. I opened up my shoulders to clip it off my legs. But the ball swung late, from leg to off. I remember readjusting my feet, realigning my shoulders and swinging through the line of the ball, sending it, like

SUPER PIECE OF CRICKET, THAT!

a bullet, if I may say so myself, to the mid-on boundary. The crowd gasped with appreciation: a classic on drive, the hardest shot in the book of cricket.

This memory is instructive. Although I remember it as I've described, I also know that this memory is *impossible* — because I simply could not have had the experience that I sincerely take myself to remember having. My guess is that the bowler's speed of delivery in miles per hour was in the region of the low eighties. Positively pedestrian for a pro, blindingly fast for a fifteen-year-old boy who had never faced anything like this before. The ball would have been in the air for around half a second before it reached me, but the ball started swinging late, well after it was halfway down the track. I would have had approximately 0.2 seconds to react. Consciousness is slow: it takes at least 0.5 seconds from the time light hits the eye for the neural message to reach the higher levels of the visual cortex where detailed, conscious representations are formed. I must, it seems, have hit the ball before the neural processes I describe could have occurred. The best-case scenario is that the memories arose a short time after the episode I decribed. But that is not the way I remember it. I remembered shifting my feet *because* I saw the ball swinging towards the off side — just *as* the ball was swinging. But that is precisely what could not have happened. We now know that the visual system is divided into two distinct tracks. My reactions were driven by the *dorsal* visual stream — the visual pathway responsible for action guidance. The *ventral* visual stream — responsible for detailed conscious awareness – wouldn't have been fast enough to keep up. Therefore, this seems to be the long and short of the matter. There was an episode. It happened in a certain way. And I might actually remember it happening in the way it actually happened. But I could not, at the time, have experienced it as happening in the way I remember it happening – even if it did happen in that way. So, what *did* happen?

As Neisser predicts, what happened was testimony, along with a not insignificant quantity of beer. Beer-fuelled, prolonged, boorish testimony. After the game I was plied with beer and asked to explain how I had played *that* shot. That's how I remember it, but I have to acknowledge that it might have been me plying myself with beer and offering largely unsolicited reminiscences of my earlier legerdemain. Whatever actually happened, these reminiscences were a way of reconstructing my memory. In working out what I must have done to hit the ball in this way, I fashioned, reshaped – reconstructed – my memory. So now I remember – sincerely – what I think I must have done, whether or not I in fact did it. This memory – if that is what it is – seems to me as real as any memory. Is it, nevertheless, a confabulation? Not in the standard sense. In a confabulation, I would seem to remember something that never really happened. But this episode did happen. And it is quite probable that it happened in the way I remember it happening. It is difficult to see how else I could have hit the ball in the way I did. Nevertheless, what I remember – or 'remember' – is my

SUPER PIECE OF CRICKET, THAT!

rational reconstruction of the episode.

Negotiation (noun): 'discussion aimed at reaching an agreement'. This process of working out the way an episode must have happened, and then remembering it in the way thus worked out, is an example of what we might think of as a *negotiation* with one's past. I discuss with myself the various things that *might* have happened and eventually agree with myself on what *must* have happened. Ultimately, I remember what I think must have happened – the version of the event that I agreed upon with myself – whether or not it really did happen this way. I negotiated with my past, and ultimately remembered the results of that negotiation. Did the past actually happen that way? Maybe. Maybe not. I remember what I think must have happened, and not necessarily what actually did happen. But if it did happen that way, then there is a clear sense in which I remember accurately. It is just that the formation of my memory has taken a somewhat idiosyncratic trajectory.

21

THE FACE OF MY FATHER, REDUX

We might think of the cricketing example as proof of the existence of a certain kind of negotiation with the past. I have a memory that seems as clear to me as most other memories. It is quite likely that the remembered episode occurred in the way it occurred: the things I remember happening and the things I remember doing may well have happened and may well have been done in the way I remember. But I know I couldn't have had the experiences I remember myself to have had of these happenings and doings at the time they happened and were done. This is an example of me having negotiated with my past. Through negotiation, I rationally reconstructed a past, and then remembered the reconstruction, not the past itself – although the former and the latter may, in fact, be the same.

If this is indeed an example of negotiation with the past,

THE FACE OF MY FATHER, REDUX

we can regard it as an instance of a more general phenomenon of negotiation, not restricted to contexts of high-velocity sport. Suppose I recall something that I have not thought about for many years. The memory of this episode, once crystal clear, has now faded, and accordingly puzzles me a little. To make sense of it I add some details pertaining to the context of the memory – for example, the circumstances that led up to it, perhaps adding details I could have known about only after the remembered episode took place. This contextualization helps me to understand why the remembered episode occurred and the way it occurred. The contextualization need not be correct, but it may well be. And whether correct or incorrect, it can be part of a process of working out how the past must have occurred and then remembering it in the way that one has thus worked out. We do not merely have memories; we make sense of them. And to this extent, remembering can often be the result of our negotiation with the past. We negotiate with the past precisely to make sense of the present, and then we often remember the results of our negotiation rather than the past itself.

Negotiation, however, is a tricky concept. Who negotiates with whom and about what is not always as clear as it seems. In more familiar negotiatory circumstances, negotiation with oneself is comparatively rare. Negotiation, typically, is between at least two different parties. The past may be one of these parties, but whether you are the other is by no means a foregone conclusion. This applies in the case of memory as much as it does anywhere else. To see why, it is time we returned to the face of my father in 1965.

I wrote that I remembered my father's face progressively transforming from confusion to suspicion to grim resignation to happiness. That is, indeed, how I remember it. The memory is as clear as any I have. But how much would the two-year-and-eight-month-old me really have understood of confusion, suspicion and grim resignation? I remember the face undergoing successive transformations from one of these states to the next. But it is doubtful to say the least that I would have – could have – experienced them as confusion, suspicion and grim resignation at that time. Yet, this is the way I now see my father's face in my memory. Why would this be?

The most obvious explanation, and, as far as I can see, the only explanation, is that my memory is really a reconstruction of the episode, driven by my father's (not infrequent) post hoc reminiscences. As I think I mentioned earlier, he wasn't about to let that go! These reminiscences would incorporate not only the bare details of what happened, but also a blow-by-blow account of what was going on in his mind as these things happened. 'At first, I thought they were showing the end of the last fight ... Then I thought, Did you fiddle with the TV or something? Then I realized the fight was over ...' And so on and so forth. The end result is that I now remember an episode as it was reconstructed by my father. I now remember what I have been told to remember: I remember what I have been told happened.

Like the cricketing memory, it is likely that this

THE FACE OF MY FATHER, REDUX

reconstruction is a memory and not a confabulation. A confabulation occurs when I seem to remember something that never really happened. But this episode, or something very like it, did happen. At least, there is evidence that points both to it happening and to it happening in more or less the way I remember it happening. My father's face may well have progressively transformed from confusion to suspicion to grim resignation to happiness. Indeed, if my father's testimony was correct, then his face would have progressively transformed in this way. On the other hand, it may not. But even if it did, I could not have experienced it in this way at that time. Therefore, I do not remember it *as* I formerly experienced it. I may well be remembering what happened, but I do not remember what happened *as* I experienced it at the time it happened. This memory has arisen out of negotiation. Like the cricketing memory, it is a memory that has arisen out of a reconstruction of the past. But in this case, the reconstruction is one supplied by my father rather than by me. The process of negotiation has spread out to incorporate my father's reconstruction of what happened. What I remember is my father's account of the episode rather than the episode as I experienced it at the time. The memory is mine. But it seems it is also his. As much his as it is mine.

22

OWNERSHIP AND AUTHORSHIP IN MEMORY

Suppose Picasso's *Le Rêve* were hanging on my living-room wall. Alas, only in my dreams, of course, but just suppose. Whose painting is this? On the one hand, I could make a case for it being mine – if, for example, I were able to point to valid documents of sale establishing that I, in fact, legally own it. The painting would then be mine by virtue of my *ownership* of it. On the other hand, Picasso has a good case for the painting being his. It is his painting as opposed to Dalí's or Braque's: it is his painting in the sense that he created it. That is, the painting is Picasso's by virtue of his *authorship* of it. These answers do not compete with one another. That they are both perfectly legitimate answers to the question of 'Whose painting is this?' shows that the question is ambiguous. A painting might be mine because of my ownership of it, or it might be mine through my authorship

OWNERSHIP AND AUTHORSHIP IN MEMORY

of it. Now we can see that the same is true of memories. For any memory you might have, there is a question of its ownership and there is another, quite distinct, question of its authorship.

The distinction between ownership and authorship of a memory provides a useful way of understanding what is going on with the memories of my father's face. His (habitual) recounting of the episode has been superimposed on my memory of that episode. In effect, I remember his recounting of the episode *as* a memory of the episode itself. Whose memory is this? Is it mine? It seems I have a good legal claim to it. I think I can make a reasonable case for claiming ownership of this memory, grounded in its being housed in my brain. My brain is housing it, and therefore I possess it. And possession, as we all know, is nine-tenths of the law. After all, this seems to be a modal truth about memory: whenever there is a memory, there is someone who has it – in the sense of owning it. As my father is no longer around to have this memory, it seems that this someone must be me. It is mine by default at the very least.

There is another, deeper sense in which I own this memory. Remember, my fingerprints are all over it. In this memory, I transformed my father's face from that of the thirty-five-year-old man he would have been when the remembered episode occurred to the face of an old man, the man of his final years. In effect, I edited this memory – precisely so that I was able to have it. Therefore, I also own this memory in the sense that I am its *editor* or *curator*.

THE BOOK OF MEMORY

Perhaps, sometimes, there is a fine line between editing and authoring a work. While acknowledging that the former can sometimes slide into the latter, I choose to think of them as distinct. The distinction may be one of degree rather than kind, and so not a firm distinction. But the absence of a firm distinction is not the absence of a distinction. (That some people are of average height – neither short nor tall – does not alter the fact that some people are short and some are tall, even though short gradually shades into tall.) Editing a memory is one way of becoming its owner. I own this memory of my father's face both because I house it in my brain and because I have edited it. Housing it in my brain would on its own be enough for ownership. But in this case, I own the memory in both senses.

What I am not, however, is the author of this memory. Authorship of this memory belongs to my father, by virtue of his interminable recounting of the episode. Every time it is recalled a memory must be reconsolidated. If it is not, it disappears. Reconsolidation is the process whereby a memory is *re-created*. My father's frequent impromptu recounting of this episode achieved two things. First, it was responsible for my retrieval of the memory, in what we now know is the soft, labile form characteristic of a memory that has been retrieved but not yet reconsolidated. Second, it helped shape the process of reconsolidation, casting the memory in a form inspired by the content of the recounting itself. My father's recounting of the episode was part of the process whereby my memory was re-created. As a result, when I recall this

OWNERSHIP AND AUTHORSHIP IN MEMORY

episode now, I am recalling a re-creation of my father. I recall his re-creation, not mine.

   The significance of this authorship becomes all the more apparent when we recall that memories, like many other mental states, are, as philosophers sometimes put it, *individuated* by their content. The memory of my father's face is a different memory from the memory of my cricketing on drive precisely because the memories are about different things. The contents of the memories are different and that is why they are different memories. Memories make us who we are. But their contents make memories what they are. You can appreciate, then, the importance of my father's creation – and indefatigable re-creations – of the content of this memory. The content of this memory has been supplied by my father. What makes the memory the memory that it is, and what differentiates it from all other memories, is something that has been supplied by my father's repeated commentary on the episode. The defining feature of the memory has been supplied not by me but by him. The memory, thus, seems to be a curious amalgam of mine and his. It is mine to the extent I am its owner. I am its owner to the extent that the memory is housed in my brain. I am its owner, also, to the extent that I have added my editorial stamp to it. But it is also my father's memory. It is his to the extent that he is its author, the creator of its content. He was the one who created this memory that now lies in my brain, and which bears my stamp, and he did so by fashioning – in my brain, no less – the content that individuates it.

THE BOOK OF MEMORY

It may seem to you that this is an especially unusual memory. But I don't think it is. The conditions that give rise to this kind of memory – where ownership and authorship are divided between two different people – are not at all uncommon. Only two conditions need to be met for this possibility to arise, and they are both relatively quotidian. The first is that one person engages in repeated – perhaps habitual – spoken externalizations of an episode. The second is that there be another person who is available to receive this commentary. The repeated commentary by the first person incites in the second person the memory's retrieval. This retrieval returns the memory to a nascent, labile form. The commentary then subsequently re-shapes the memory in the form suggested by the first person's commentary. These sorts of circumstances are common ones, almost inevitably arising when two people spend much of their lives together.

Just as in the case of the painting, there is no real answer to the question, 'Whose memory is this?' If I were the owner of *Le Rêve*, Picasso would still be its author. Similarly, it seems I am the owner of this memory, and my father is its author. All we can do in response to the question of whose memory it is – *really* – is point out these facts of ownership and authorship. There is ownership and there is authorship, and there is nothing more basic than that. Memories are owned and they are authored, and the owner of any given memory is not always the same person as the author.

23

MIRACLES

Let us take a moment to bask in the warm, rosy glow of the miracle I have just described. Those who have gone, we sometimes say, live on in our memories. How much of a consolation this is to those who have gone, or to those who are about to go, is unclear. Consolation or not, we all understand the idea of the departed living on in our memories. That is not what I am talking about.

My father does live on in many of my memories. But these are *my* memories. Both owned and authored by me. The memory of the face of my father in 1965 is not my memory. At least, it has as much claim to being my father's memory as it has to being mine. It is my memory to the extent that it is housed in my brain. It is my memory, also, to the extent that (a) I remember an episode in my past, (b) this episode happened, and (c) I experience it as an episode I formerly encountered – a result achieved via a little editorial endeavour on my part: I have transformed the age of my father's face,

THE BOOK OF MEMORY

and I have done this precisely so I can remember this face as the face of my father. However, it is my father's memory to the extent that I never experienced the episode in the way I now remember it. Only he experienced the episode in the way I remember it. I remember, in other words, a series of events related to me by my father rather than the experiences I had at the time these events took place. The memory I now have is the result of a negotiation with the past that my father made but that I never did. This memory is, therefore, not wholly my father's, and neither is it wholly mine. The memory is an elusive combination of his and mine.

We might put the point this way. My father is responsible for *what* is remembered. But I am responsible for the *way* in which it is remembered. My father is responsible for the *content* of the memory: what the memory says. The memory says that on a certain day long ago, at the time of an athletic confrontation with an unexpectedly abrupt conclusion, the face of my father progressively transformed from confusion to suspicion to resignation to happiness. My father's post hoc reminiscences are responsible for the memory saying this. But I am responsible for transforming the face into the face of his later, final years, a transformation wrought precisely so I might remember this episode. We might think of this as the memory's *style*: the way it says what it says. My father is responsible for the content of the memory, thus qualifying the memory as his. But I am at least partly responsible for the style of the memory, thus qualifying the memory as mine.

Any book is an amalgam of content and style, of what it

MIRACLES

says and the way it says it. But content can, in principle, come from anywhere. The content of this memory of my father's face comes from my father, not from me. Others may similarly insert sentences into the book of me. But if they do, I will then add my own twist to these, precisely so they may find a suitable home in my book. The book's style is ineluctably mine. Style is essential to me, to who I am, in a way that content can never be. My father's memory found a place in a new home, in my mind, in the book of me. What makes this new home a suitable one, a home where my father's memory might flourish, is its ability to transform episodes in a certain way – precisely so that these episodes may be remembered. An episode remembered by my father is given my own distinctive twist. And this twist is added precisely so that I can remember it too. My father's frequent post hoc reminiscences of the episode provide the content of the memory. The memory's content comes from my father. But on this content, I have imposed a style. The memory is an amalgam of content and style, and therefore also an amalgam of his memory and mine.

Nevertheless, the memory is, in part, my father's memory. To the extent that my father lives on in this memory, he is living on through *his* memory as much as through mine. On the face of it, this seems to be a more robust sense of living on. His memories were supposed to be what made my father the person he was. My memories don't make him the person he was. Only his memories did that. But now we find, living on in me, one of his memories, or a memory that has as much right to be regarded as his as it does to be regarded as mine. Something that helped make him who he was lives on. A constituent of my father has found its way into my mind and set up home there. This might be far more consoling to my father – if he were around to be consoled – than simply living on in my memories. Seemingly unimpeded by his death, this memory that is partly his endures. My father lives on in my memories. But more importantly, he also lives on in his memories.

There is more to your survival than living on in the memories of others. It is not simply that you exist in their memories. Your memories – or, at least, things that are partly your memories – themselves can endure. You can live on in your memories too. Memories make us who we are. Thus, something that made you who you were can live on in someone else, long after you have gone, partly making them who they are too. There is therefore more to your life than can be contained within the temporal parameters of your birth and death. There is more to your life than can be constrained by the spatial boundaries of your body. We are messy creatures, with little respect for boundaries, recognizing that these are always mutable. We people are porous; we are permeable. What you are – your essence – can bleed out of you into a time long after you are dead. What you are can bleed out into the fabric of others. The question of when and where you begin and when and where you end has no straightforward answer.

24

SO LONG, SUCKERS!

I once had a distant cousin or uncle, his name now forgotten, who I never saw much. That's the way my father's half of the family was. For the last twenty-five years of his life, I don't think my father talked to his brother, John – not even once. This was not, as far as I know, because they had any kind of falling out, but because they simply couldn't think of anything to say to each other. With my cousin (or uncle), I seem to remember there had been some sort of disagreement with my father concerning the circumstances in which one may legitimately castle in chess, a crime deserving of lifelong exile if ever there was one. I never saw him after that. Years later, I remember my grandmother – my father's mother, Nana Christchurch as we knew her, since we identified our grandparents by where they resided – talking about him over lunch in our house one day: 'Well, at least someone in this family turned out right.'

'What the bloody hell are you talking about?' one of us said. I

THE BOOK OF MEMORY

don't remember who said it, but it certainly sounds like my dad.

'Well, you know, going to these places, spreading the word of God...'

She thought he was a missionary. He was, in fact, a mercenary, who died in West Africa, or so I seem to remember being told. A kinder family would presumably have allowed this elderly woman, not far from death, to hold on to this comforting illusion. Our family, on the other hand, was a different kind of beast.

Why do I tell you this? Simply because I have never seen my family laugh, en bloc – minus poor Nana – as much, or as wholeheartedly, as we did then. This is one of the best memories I have. If there is the prospect of any of my memories living on after I have gone, I definitely want to try to give this memory every chance of being one of them. My sons have heard the story a few times already, and I am going to keep repeating it until they start constructing images, detailed memoryscapes, of the grandmother they never met being mercilessly taunted by her kin, most of whom are now gone. One day, if all goes to plan, it will seem to them as if they were there.

That's the thing about us old folks. You think we keep repeating things because we are losing our marbles. That may be true some or most of the time. But we do it also as a means of survival. It is our memories that we are deftly sending in the direction of your brain, hoping they will set up home there. The home I have provided my memories with, currently three score years plus change, is slowly, but undeniably, becoming non-viable. It's not up to code anymore,

SO LONG, SUCKERS!

I am sure. A new home is needed for my memories. Any memory is potentially a parasite, you know.

In the days after I have gone, my sons, you will have memories of me. How many of these are yours and how many are mine, and the precise balance of you and me in each of them, will be a matter of often complex interpretation. Think back on the times we had together, and on how I would encourage you to remember those times, talking fondly of them. Think of the photographs I made you look at on *Snapfish*, photographs that captured times when you were small and, more to the point, impressionable. Think of how I explained to you what was going on in these mementos of times *perdu*. Where we were, where we had been, what we were doing, where we were going, and much more besides. A classic study in reconsolidation. Someone of a cynical bent might ask themselves a question. Could it really be that I was negotiating your past for you? Could it really be that I was trying to ensure my own survival – or some facsimile of my own survival – by planting my memories in your heads, so that my memories would live on with your memories, existing together side by side, cheek by jowl, long after I was gone? I confess: even I do not know the answer to this question. But it's something for you to think about. So long, suckers! Yours truly, Dad.

Postface

MY AFTERLIFE AS A FICTIONAL CHARACTER

Our understanding of fiction is an instructive example of our habit of ignoring what is most important in favour of what is most obvious. The most obvious feature of fiction – its untruth – is not its most important. The essence of fiction is to be found in the dependent existence, and the resulting incompleteness, of fictional characters. When a real human dies, his being finally becomes fixed. It congeals into a solid mass. Everything he ever was and everything he would ever become is now determined once and for all, with no further additions or subtractions to this being possible. He now is what he was, and will never again be anything more than that. Such is the destiny of the ontically rotund, or so it is commonly thought.

On the other hand, a fictional human, such as Sherlock Holmes, is ontically thin. This means that the being of such a character is essentially dependent on others. There is no fact of the matter concerning what Holmes did on the morning of 24 April 1888 unless someone, Conan Doyle or his fanfiction inheritors, has written this somewhere and at some time. The being of Holmes, the type of existence possessed by Holmes, is, in this sense, dependent on others. His existence is a dependent existence. For this very reason, his being is always essentially unfinished. His existence is essentially dependent on what others write – and who knows what or when others are going to write – to add to his being in manners of their devising. Holmes's being, even in principle, cannot be completed. That is why Holmes, like all fictional characters, can never definitively die. An existence that cannot be completed is an existence that can never end.

I have tried to convince you that this simple division between the real, as we tendentiously put it, and the fictional is, while largely true, not entirely so. There is a point where the borderline between the real and the fictional frays, wears thin, and where the distinction between the inhabitants of each realm is at its most attenuated. This region of existential porosity is made up of memories. Memory is where the boundary between reality and fiction comes most under pressure – sometimes, perhaps, approaching the point of rupture.

It is in our memories that we most closely approximate fictional characters. This is not because our memories are false or otherwise fictional, although they are likely to be to varying degrees inaccurate, especially in their episodicity. The endemic falsity of memories does not matter. It's obvious, but

MY AFTERLIFE AS A FICTIONAL CHARACTER

ultimately rather unimportant. What is important is that, paradoxically, in my memories – the very memories that make me who I am – I am at my ontologically most ambiguous. When a memory is recalled, it must be completed anew. A new draft must be written. Every memory upon retrieval calls out to be completed. This demand is insistent, and if it is not satisfied the memory fades into nothingness.

So strident is the call for completion that memory is more than willing to turn a blind eye to the identity of who answers this call. My memories are typically completed by me, every time I retrieve them. But there is nothing, in principle, that rules out their being completed by others. A memory summoned from the void must return to soft and pliable form. It will re-harden, but the specific form this re-hardening takes, the specific content captured in its newly hardened form, can depend on others as much as it can on me. Each new hardening of a memory thus summoned is a negotiation with the past, but who drives this negotiation is always an open question.

The result, as we have seen, is that a memory authored and originally owned by one person can come to be owned by another if that other is willing and able to rewrite it, and so complete it. In this way, memories authored by one person can eventually find their way into the minds of others. Memories authored by my father live on in me, their new owner. It may be that one day memories authored by me will live on in my sons. If so, I will survive in these memories that are, at least partly, mine.

THE BOOK OF MEMORY

It's true that this is a survival that many will find wanting – those, that is, whose conception of survival is decisively shaped by a certain attitude highlighted in the Hindu–Buddhist tradition – namely, *upādāna*, the attitude of holding tight, of clinging, to the person you think you are. Survival of death grounded in *upādāna* emphasizes continuity, the preservation of you in your entirety, or of some essential part or aspect of you. In the West, this has engendered certain specific pictures of survival such as the continuation of an immortal soul or the resurrection of the body on Judgement Day. I, on the other hand, have always been an advocate of *moksha*, of letting go, recognizing that there was really never anything there to which one might cling.

Je est un autre, as the poet Arthur Rimbaud once put it. I is another. I is somebody else, if only in part. The memories of others have become mine, owned if not authored by me. That which helped make my father the person he was now plays the same role in me. People are like that. We overlap. We are porous beings, rather than impermeable substances that exist essentially independently of each other. The boundaries between us are not fixed but shifting. Sometimes these boundaries are thin and delicate. Sometimes they barely exist at all. We are all, each one of us, many somebodies.

This, then, is my hope for the future. My memories are going on a journey. They are going on it with you, my sons. These memories have helped make me who I am. You have taken them in, given them a home, and added your own little

MY AFTERLIFE AS A FICTIONAL CHARACTER

editorial twists, and they will now play a role in making you who you are. In some respects, I am like Sherlock Holmes. My being is no longer my own, but rests on your retrieval and subsequent rewriting. My existence will now be a dependent one, and therefore incompletable. But an incompletable existence can never end. An incompletable being can never die. Our memories make us immortal, even when we are no longer around to have them. In other respects, I am like Conan Doyle. I authored these memories that are now owned by you. Nothing can change that. Owned by you, authored by me: where these memories exist, the boundaries between us are gossamer thin. It is not possible for us to be any closer than this, my sons. Where these memories are, the distance between us dwindles to nothing, and, inseparable, we venture on into a future as yet undetermined. Perhaps you would have preferred that I bequeathed to you Ferraris rather than these curious memories, both mine and yours. I wouldn't blame you. But for me, you should know, this may be the most exciting thing that has ever happened.

FURTHER READING

Preface: My Life as a Fictional Character

The Tennessee Williams play referred to is *The Milk Train Doesn't Stop Here Anymore* (1963).

'All your piety and wit cannot call it back to cancel half a line.' This is from Edward FitzGerald's, *The Rubáiyát of Omar Khayyám* (1859).

Plato's attitude towards writing can be found in his *Phaedrus*.

Part One: The Book of Memory

Ludwig Wittgenstein's remark that a philosophical question 'has the form: I don't know my way about', and his remarks on the nature of philosophy more generally, can be found in his posthumously published *Philosophical Investigations* (1953).

THE BOOK OF MEMORY

The necessity of origin is an idea strongly associated with the philosopher Saul Kripke. See, in particular, his book *Naming and Necessity* (1980).

I was made aware of the proverb *Einmal ist keinmal* through Milan Kundera's incomparable *The Unbearable Lightness of Being* (1984), where the proverb features as one of the book's motifs.

The distinction between semantic and episodic memory was first drawn in Endel Tulving's groundbreaking paper, 'Episodic and semantic memory', *Organization of Memory* (1972). The concept of autonoesis was also introduced in this paper.

The case of R.B. is discussed in Stan Klein and Shaun Nichols, 'Memory and the sense of personal identity', *Mind* (2012).

The first published work on SDAM was in Palombo et al., 'Severely deficient autobiographical memory (SDAM) in healthy adults: a new mnemonic syndrome', *Neuropsychologia* (2015).

The first published work on HSAM is LePort et al., 'Behavioral and neuroanatomical investigation of Highly Superior Autobiographical Memory (HSAM),' *Neurobiology of Learning and Memory* (2012).

FURTHER READING

Part Two: The Waters of Lethe

Coleridge's ruminations on memory can be found in his *Notebooks* (1803). Bergson's views can be found in his *Matter and Memory* (1896[1908]).

The passage from Rilke is from his *Notebooks of Malte Laurids Brigge* (1910). I introduce the idea of what I christen 'Rilkean memory' in my book *Memory and the Self* (2017).

Bachelard's view on what I call 'embodied Rilkean memory' can be found in his excellent book *The Poetics of Space* (1958).

Aharon Appelfeld's example of a form of memory that involves both embodied and affective constituents is taken from his *Story of a Life* (1999).

Nietzsche's famous aphorism is found in his book *The Joyful Wisdom* (1882), Section 290.

Part Three: Bright Islands in the Night

With a delightfully unfussy writing style, Beyle/Stendhal's work is always worth a visit. The discussion here is based on the juxtaposition of his accounts given in his (1817/1826) book *Rome, Naples and Florence* and his *Private Journals* of

1811. My attention was first drawn to this juxtaposition by Julian Barnes in his excellent *Nothing to be Frightened of* (2009).

The classic statement of the 'flashbulb memory' hypothesis can be found in R. Brown and J. Kulik, 'Flashbulb memories', *Cognition* (1977).

Neisser and Harsch's classic study of the *Challenger* explosion can be found in their 'Phantom flashbulbs: false recollections of hearing the news about *Challenger*', in Winograd & Neisser (Eds), *Affect and Accuracy in Recall: Studies of 'Flashbulb' Memories* (1992).

Karim Nader's groundbreaking work on the significance of reconsolidation can be found in his 'Memory traces unbound', *Trends in Neurosciences* (2003).

Todd Sacktor's discovery about the relevance of protein PKMzeta is recorded in 'Memory maintenance by PKMζ: an evolutionary perspective,' *Molecular Brain* (2012).

Plato's theory of memory is presented in his *Theaetetus*. Augustine's storehouse model is presented in his *Confessions*.

For a good study of the phenomena of field and observer memories, see Chris McCarroll, *Remembering from the Outside: Personal Memory and the Perspectival Mind* (2018).

FURTHER READING

Part Four: Negotiating with the Past

Neisser's study of memories of the 1989 California earthquake can be found in his 'Remembering the earthquake: direct experience vs. hearing the news', *Memory* (1996).

Nietzsche's famous epigram can be found in his *Beyond Good and Evil* (1886), chapter 4.

I have been wrestling with this memory of my father's face for some years. Every time I return to it, I find more in it, and I hope to be at least asymptotically approaching completeness in my account now. An earlier – inadequate – attempt to grapple with it, and with some of these issues more generally, can be found in my book *Memory and the Self* (2017).

ACKNOWLEDGEMENTS

I have been thinking about the ideas in this book for some years. It all started with a photograph, of two canids, a wolf hybrid and a dog, charging around Inchydoney beach in County Cork, Ireland, probably somewhere around 1997. What was significant about this photograph was the teeth marks left in it by a third party, Tess, a wolfdog who wasn't even born at the time the scene depicted in this photograph occurred. The coin dropped – rather slowly, I have to admit. In addition to the content of the photograph – what it is about – the photograph also has a style, in this case a raggedy style born of Tess's masticatory efforts. This style is not essentially tethered to the time of the photograph's content, but it helps shape that content. This, for me, gradually evolved into a template for thinking about memory, and it informs many of the central ideas of this book. So: thank you, Tess!

My thanks to the College of Arts and Sciences at the University of Miami for providing me with valuable support during the researching and writing of this book. My greatest thanks, as always, are to my family: to my wife Emma and my sons Brenin and Macsen.